the
Mama Bamba
way

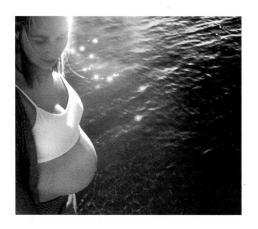

The power and pleasure
of natural childbirth

BY ROBYN SHELDON
PHOTOGRAPHY BY NIKKI RIXON

FINDHORN PRESS

First published in South Africa in 2008
by Sharp Sharp Media

This updated edition first published in the rest of the word in 2010
by Findhorn Press

ISBN: 978-1-84409-189-8

Design and layout: Adéle Sherlock

Published by
Findhorn Press
117-121 High Street,
Forres IV36 1AB, Scotland, UK
t +44(0)1309 690582
f +44(0)131 777 2711
e info@findhornpress.com
www.findhornpress.com

CONTENTS

For Rory, Maf, and Nix,
who taught me a lot about birth,
and even more about love.

The Mama Bamba Way

" Learn from mothers and babies; every one of them has a unique story to tell. Look for wisdom in the humblest places—that's usually where you'll find it. "

— *Lois Wilson, American midwife* [1]

In Botswana, the weaver birds made nests in the garden every spring. The males had bright yellow chests and were devoted to the task. Nest building was a laborious construction of twigs, grass, feathers, cotton waste from my bin in the barn, bits of thatch from the eaves and, most loved of all, threads from my banana palm, which never fully recovered from its annual spring shredding.

Each material was carefully selected for its particular properties of sturdiness, flexibility, softness, or its ability to withstand the harsh Botswana climate. The weaving may not always have been as neat as their mate's high standards of excellence required, but eventually they created homes for their fledglings and kept them safe, for a while at least, from snakes, birds of prey, and the scorching sun.

This book is weaving of a different type, so many different strands from my life experiences coming together here to gradually grow an idea about how to birth with love.

My meditation practice forms the skeleton strand of the book. Twenty years of daily sitting have given me an understanding of the tremendous power of staying in the moment, of simply being with the substance of whatever is presenting itself right now. In birth there is no more valuable attitude that we can bring to the task than simply being with it. This supports the process, helps the cervix to dilate without resistance, and I strongly intuit that it might also help the baby to adjust to its life outside the womb.

My meditation practice has taught me to appreciate not only spiritual wisdom, which grows imperceptibly over long periods and is a palpable quality in some of my wonderful spiritual teachers, but also to embrace the indelicate stuff of our everyday existence. I have developed the deepest respect for delicious chocolate and warm nourishing soup, for baby's first cries, for the tearing asunder of a mother's heart at a miscarriage, for Sunday lie-ins, for e-mails from my children, for the river next to my house wildly careering around corners in flood and crashing through new bulbs planted too lovingly close to its edges, for broccoli and beans. Those beans from the children's chant: "Beans, beans are good for your heart / The more you eat, the more you fart / The more you fart the better you feel / So eat your beans at every meal."

In other words, I have developed respect for life itself, including the ghastly newspaper reminder this morning of child rape in our suburbs. This meditation practice supports me to respect life in its glory and its hardships and that, I have discovered, is a very good approach to have at a birth.

The next thread of the weaving is supplied from the Integration Therapy I studied with Marlies van Boxtel in the Netherlands. Marlies is a Jungian psychoanalyst who was taught Integration Therapy for eight years by spiritual healer and visionary Chris Griscom in Santa Fe, New Mexico. In Santa Fe they are called "Light Institute Intensives." For years before training as a midwife, I used Integration Therapy to work with clients on deeper levels of consciousness and with the symbolic stories that are held there, which subtly mold and direct our external life experiences. This therapy has become invaluable in my work with pregnant women, enriching their births and facilitating a deeper relationship with their unborn babies.

The counseling thread that derived from training with Hospice and Lifeline drew me to midwifery practice as a career. Birth and death each have a sacred quality about them that is experienced intensely when we allow them to show themselves through being present to their timelessness. My own births taught me this initially, and I recognized a similar feeling with the Hospice work, so I went in search of that quality of attention as part of my clients' birth experiences.

There's the thread of encouraging a deepening of trance states during labor. This thread can be teased out into deriving from different sources: San dances in the Kalahari as a young woman, Sangoma tribal dances later in life, meditation practice again, HypnoBirthing—a technique of deep relaxation in which I trained in the United States, Biodanza dance classes for awakening our vitality and life force, or the gentle trance of simply sitting quietly in the mountains sometimes. All these threads come together at birth to encourage women to surrender into that trance place that is the natural home of labor. The less resistance a woman has to going deep within herself and surrendering to the labor, the more likely her body is to open to birthing without a struggle.

The thread of using art as a tool for pregnant women to find out more about themselves and their relationships with their babies, and as one more way to enjoy their pregnancy, came from my original career as a university graduate in art and as a ceramicist. I am not surprised, in retrospect, that I chose ceramics as my major subject. It was the pit, wood, and raku firings that drew me to it. The same sense of patience, and of simply being there tending the fire or the kiln, is what appeals to me about tending women in labor. It's a soft time of receptivity and quiet—of careful watching to decide when to throw another log of wood on the fire, which is so similar to watching when to encourage a birth partner's support or when to wipe a mother's brow during her labor.

Then finally, there's the physiological thread of midwifery. Built up slowly over painstaking years of poring over midwifery and obstetric texts for distance learning exams in the United States, of practical tutorials and long hours of night duties at the mission hospital in Ramotswa, of bureaucratic red tape and endless obstacles to certification, and ultimately, of many fulfilling hours attending women wherever they felt most at home giving birth to their babies.

Each thread on its own might make a thin and uncomfortable or unsupportive nest for a woman in labor, but laced together and each woven into its correct place they lend richness to this nest, which can assist women to trust their bodies and to feel held by its embrace.

In the same way that mind and body are interdependent, or that the food we eat cannot be separated from the sun, the rain, the earth, and the seed that created it, so my colleagues and clients form an integral part of this nest. At **Mama Bamba**, I work together with Justine Evans, a clinical psychologist, to provide a supportive place for women to prepare for birth. **Mama Bamba** is a place where women explore their pregnant environment and their birth choices through using movement, mindful awareness, relaxation, dance, toning, and art. Most importantly, it is a meeting place for women to exchange ideas, become inspired, and play with their beliefs about pregnancy, birth, and parenting.

The Mama Bamba Way describes the potential we have as women to transform our lives, our self images, and our babies' perceptions of the world through birthing with integrity and awareness. It contains the processes and techniques I encourage women to explore pre-birth that can support them in their labor, so that no matter how it unfolds, birth is a satisfying experience for them. There are as many tools for labor as there are paths up a mountain—these are simply some of the ones we use at Mama Bamba, although we continuously add new ones in an organic process of growth. The core tools are those of meditative awareness, relaxation, and surrender, deep exploration of our unconscious processes, connecting with our babies in the womb and labor support.

This book also includes guidance for labor, practical advice for the early months of parenting, and what to do when we suffer from the loss of a baby, pre- or post-birth. Although it is an uncommon event, it is included here because it remains unaddressed and avoided too much in our society.

I have also included birth stories, both from women I've worked with and from those who have crossed my path and offered me their stories to enrich my life. Birthing women have a wealth of stories about their experiences. Many of these women are empowered by their birth experiences. Their stories illustrate the potential we hold within us to give birth in an authentic and committed way. They illustrate our ability to surrender to the birthing process, because by doing so, we are initiated into a wiser and more empowered way of being women. The birth preparation section details many of the tools employed by the women who have generously described their birth experiences throughout the book.

The Mama Bamba Way - **Guided Relaxation for Birth CD** is available from publisher Findhorn Press as downloadable mp3 tracks. Guided Visualizations by Robyn Sheldon – Music and Mastering by Indidginus. It features the following tracks:

GUIDED VISUALIZATION & MUSIC

1. Body Relaxation (10:37)

2. Imagining your Favorite Place (10:08)

3. Connectiong to the Free (10:12)

4. Awareness of the Child (12:00)

MUSIC

5. Dawn (9:45)

6. Daylight (9:07)

7. Twilight (9:30)

8. Night (9:10)

go to **www.findhornpress.com** and search for Robyn Sheldon or *The Mama Bamba Way*

THE POWER OF BIRTH

Chapter One

" Our deepest fear is not that we are inadequate.
Our deepest fear is that we are powerful beyond measure.
It is our light, not our darkness, that most frightens us.
We ask ourselves. Who am I to be brilliant, gorgeous,
talented, and fabulous?
Actually, who are you not to be?
You are a child of God.
Your playing small does not serve the world.
There is nothing enlightened about shrinking
so that other people will not feel insecure around you.
We were born to make manifest the glory of God that is within us.
It is not just in some of us, it is in everyone.
And as we let our own light shine, we unconsciously give others
permission to do the same.
As we are liberated from our own fear,
our presence automatically liberates others. "

— *Marianne Williamson, Author, lecturer, and spiritual activist* [2]

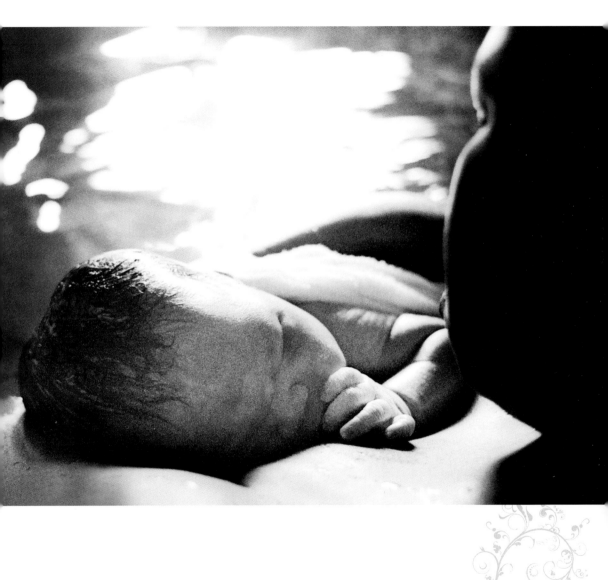

Feeling the power of birth

Anna was in tears when she was only one centimeter (0.394 inches) dilated in labor with her first child. Her cervix was rigid, she wasn't coping with her contractions, and we all secretly wondered if this might go on all night and all of the next day, too. In fact, unbeknownst to her, her contractions weren't even that strong yet.

Over the course of the next hour she slowly settled into her labor and stopped resisting the pain she was experiencing. It was awe-inspiring to notice the change in her as she surrendered into her birthing power. Her breathing deepened, she moved into a sensuous rhythm of swinging her hips back and forth on the birth ball, while her head was buried in her husband's chest. She commented cheerfully at one stage that this was easy now, and in retrospect mentioned that she had loved this stage of labor, despite the fact that her surges were clearly stronger now. She visualized her cervix opening and had a sensation of it responding to the images. Three quarters of an hour after she moved into this new pattern of labor she stood up to get into the birth pool, only to be overwhelmed with a pushing urge that was so strong that her baby was born ten minutes later. Her baby had a small smile on his face within half an hour of birth, and he and Anna are so deeply in love that, four weeks later, her intellectual capacity is still soft and squidgy.

Birth happens best through placing more awareness on our hearts than in our heads. For each birth or parenting choice, small or large, a useful question to ask is "Will this lead to more love? Or less love?" Letting go into embracing life just as it is, while taking clear, unhurried steps to change what is not harmonious, leads to more love; fighting, railing, and wailing, or avoiding life's experiences leads to less love. Birth is a time of profound experiences, whose intensity creates the ability to love more deeply.

Loving birth is a parallel experience to loving life. We cannot experience a birth filled with love and laughter without embracing the fullness of it. The idea of embracing the pain and the intensity of birth may seem frightening or foolish at first, but wholeheartedly diving into the experience transmutes it. In birth, welcoming each painful sensation as it arises has the potential to change that experience.

The interdependence of physiological, psychological, intellectual, and spiritual approaches to life is clearly exemplified at times of birth and death. These transitional states embody an intensity that, when embraced, transform us and the world around us. Birth can become ecstatic and pleasurable when we love it. Death, too, when held close, has the potential to heal enormous emotional wounds in both the dying and the grieving.

I have been at the bedside of a friend dying of cancer, who was thrashing around in a coma. As bystanders we all looked at one another helplessly, feeling out of our depth, not knowing how to help him in his terrified isolation. Then we spoke to his body, not really believing that he was anywhere that could hear us. We told it that we loved him—loved him enough to allow him to leave when the time was right. There and then he gentled and quietened, finally slipping away after four tranquil hours, with a peaceful smile on his face.

The only tool we need for embracing life, birth, or death is to trust in our body's inherent ability to love. As a midwife I know the body's incredible ability to birth naturally and to surrender to the process of birth, like an animal. From my own births, I knew the difference between fighting the pain of the contractions or staying open to the extraordinary strength of my body as wave after laboring wave surged through me. Fighting the pain created waves of fear, nausea, and excruciation. Staying open to the process was no less physically intense. But the experience was entirely different.

I am reminded of how we as women can experience sex as the most extreme pleasure or most intense pain that we know. How we perceive the sexual act is created by a multitude of factors, such as what we feel about our sexual partner, previous sexual encounters we may have had, childhood sexual abuse, fear of sex, and so on. The physical act of sex will have an impact on our perception of whether it is painful or pleasurable, but not as much as our emotional receptivity or resistance to the sex does.

Sex that we have no desire for or resist is usually an extremely painful, horribly traumatic encounter; childbirth that is feared and resisted can be equally harrowing, although the shock of it is tempered by the baby we receive as compensation for our pains. The difference is that childbirth doesn't need to be so disturbing; the fear that has built up around giving birth naturally arises out of a misconception in the collective unconscious that grew out of thousands of years of believing birth to be dirty, impure, dangerous, and primitive.

In most cultures today we think of childbirth as a purely asexual phenomenon. If we associate it with sex, it brings up ingrained taboos about incest and our own mothers. These taboos are the monsters living deep within our limbic brains, and to descend into the power of birth is to invite the monsters to show their true faces. This dark place within us may be likened to the seat of our soul. To become fully immersed in the experience of birth we need to experience our spirituality in an embodied and earthy form. When we experience spirituality in a transcendent form we feel it as universal consciousness. Spirit then is light and pure; it carries with it a calm peacefulness, a transcendence from earthly concerns. At birth we can experience our spirituality in a more matter-of-fact way if we move out of the realm of pure spirit and into the realm of our individual souls. Soul, as opposed to spirit, shows its face when we fall headlong into life. It descends into the density of life, of love, of

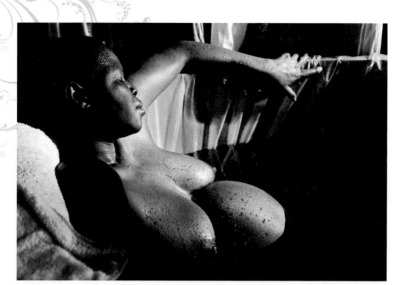

**Birth is an empowering experience for a woman,
that helps to mold her identity of herself.**

lust, of all our earthiness. When we birth within our primal knowing and our power, we are fully immersed in our soulfulness, in our raw selves, in a potent life force that embraces all of who we are, the purity and the dark places.

A powerful birth experience changes us so that we relate differently to the world around us; we are no longer sweet and kind and acceptable. It is a primal phenomenon and our fear of birth rises unbidden from its depths; not only the expected fears of pain or of dying, but also the mysterious fear of our own power. A birthing woman flings off clothes, masks, social inhibitions, and any concept of what others may think of her when she sinks into her primal birthing power. No wonder then that women choose to birth in hospitals, protected from their powerful source energy by epidurals and interventions.

As women we know how to embody our spirituality, to discover the Divine in the earth and in this dense material realm in which we live. To embody means to bring into form, to incarnate, to actualize. Over centuries women have traditionally explored the spiritual through the mundane: in tasks such as childbearing, nurturing children and gardens, washing the dishes, baking cookies. Men, on the other hand, have traditionally explored spirituality in intellectual arenas as priests, poets, and philosophers. Clearly, women with education and acknowledgement are capable of the great spiritual insights uncovered in intellectual and meditative pursuits, but it is sad if in doing so, we lose our ability to nourish the Divine in our everyday existence.

We are enriched when we reclaim the wholeness of birth. The word "holy" derives from "hal" meaning "whole, healthy, unhurt" in Middle English. Embracing the wholeness, including the intense and physical sensuality of birth, brings the sacredness back into birthing. I have assisted women who birth calmly, breathing through each surge with no resistance to the forces pouring through their body. And I have assisted women who bellow to the moon and become like Amazons as the power of the birth rushes through them. Each of these women was true to herself and responding moment by moment to the process of birth.

Women who are extremely confident and sure of themselves and their ability to surrender into their birth power may choose to birth with as little intervention as possible, occasionally even choosing to birth alone to really connect to their primitive nature. Most women choose to have a support system in place to help and encourage them with this surrender: a midwife, a partner, a mother, a birth attendant (doula), or an obstetrician. A birth companion or doula's role at a birth is to understand each individual birthing woman's needs and to respond appropriately, thus helping her to feel secure and trusting enough during birth to fully submit to the primal power of her birthing body.

There is something truly naked about the experience of a powerful birth. It is undiluted; seldom perfect in its unfolding, there may even be moments when the intensity seems overwhelming. It is also a peak life experience, with detailed memories that become deeply etched in the psyche—of a face cloth held against a cheek; a kettle glinting on the kitchen counter; a midwife's supportive hand creating counter-pressure on the sacrum; of the interior deepness of facing demons; of soft waves washing through, carrying us away, and strong ones forcing us back.

This journey is undertaken together with our babies. Their first imprints then carry the knowledge that they are not alone. Being fully present at birth is the most important gift we can give our children—if we don't fear birth, they have no reason to fear life; we bestow on them the ability to immerse themselves fully in its wonders and richness.

Sacred birth

Luna is nine months pregnant. Her body is sending labor preparation signals, and the birth is imminent. She is also a psychologist with a thriving practice, yet she has created the time to really enjoy her pregnancy. She says, "I've been much more aware of everything during the pregnancy, even nature's temperature changes or the blue sky. Everything is much brighter than normal—more beautiful, I think. I'm in a very grateful state most of the time. It was my dream that when the time was right to fall pregnant, I would be available for my child, even before the birth.

"I speak of her by her name, Laynee, which means 'God's blessings poured out". This perfectly expresses what the pregnancy has been like for me. There are always blessings around us, only sometimes they're not manifesting. This pregnancy has been like a huge jug of blessings being poured over me. There's a deep connectedness between Laynee and myself, even though she's a separate individual with her own identity and own soul. In fact, I'm more connected to her because I see her as someone coming through me, who is not me. We're on a journey together."

During pregnancy, if we give ourselves time and attention, we can become enormously peaceful, feeling linked to our babies and to a larger consciousness or oneness out of which our babies are beginning to emerge. We develop a connection with our babies beyond the simple sharing of blood, oxygen, and nourishment. Consciously or not, pregnant mothers and their babies are interdependent, and it often takes a while for this entwining of two souls to unravel into separate individuals after birth. Complementary therapists, who understand this interdependence, will sometimes, in the months after the birth, treat the mother in order to effect a change in the baby.

When we work together with our babies during the labor we can create a sacred birth experience. Babies whose mothers are consciously aware of the connection between them during the labor and birth are more likely to be alert and peaceful. When caregivers forget this and remove mothers from the intensity of their labors with epidurals and elective Caesarean sections, their babies are effectively left to experience birth unsupported by their emotional connection to their mothers. As a result of technology and medical interventions, the intense, private states of transition from woman to mother and from fetus to newborn can be overlooked, and we have become desensitized to the emotions surrounding the birth experience.

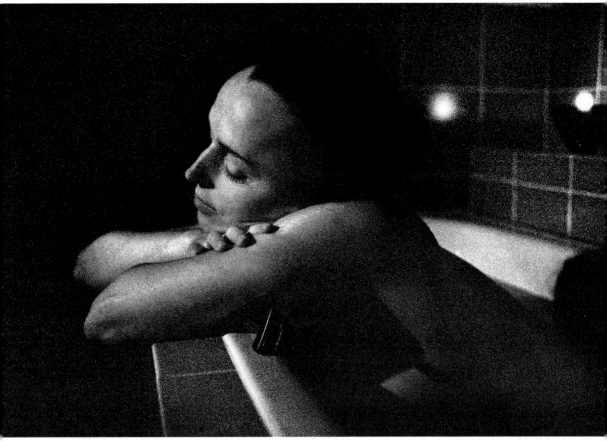

There was a palpable quality of sacredness permeating Janet's labor.

Part of the reason we often try to escape the experience of birth is because of the fear that has built up around labor. This fear arises not only from centuries of cultural condition- ing but also from television, from horror birth stories, and from the medical establishment itself; so for many women, avoiding the vivid and passionate intensity of labor is a logical choice. Society's fear and ignorance has limited the range of options available for how we give birth, sometimes to the extent that women are led to believe that a naturally born baby is not possible or even desirable. Instead of dealing with the source of the problem—fear— the medical profession worldwide expends vast sums of energy and finance on removing birth from its raw and primal state. In this process they disempower women by focusing more attention on the machines monitoring them than on the women themselves.

The input of effort required to allay fears and change the system is vast, and in South Africa, where midwives are grossly underpaid and overworked, it would be impossible for them to give more than they are already giving, while obstetricians are trained within a system that teaches them to always be on the lookout for the worst case scenarios, and to know how to deal with them. That is an obstetrician's job, and may we be forever grateful to them for taking care of those high-risk cases. Too much focus on what can go wrong with birth, however, can cause problems like fetal distress, which then require interventions, and it does distract from the awesome miracle of the birth itself.

Birth awareness is subtle. The smallest difference in attitudes and intentions about how we'll be receiving our babies can make an enormous difference to how we labor and to how they settle into this world. Babies feel more than we consciously recognize and birth psychology supports the hypothesis that a baby is wise and sensitive. Many perinatal psychologists agree that a birth can influence a baby's attitude to life, either in a positive or a negative way.

How then, do we create sacred births that can support our babies? They sometimes occur in bedrooms at home, sometimes in busy labor wards, occasionally in the operating theater with a Caesarean section. They usually occur with women who are well informed and have made a conscious choice to be part of the decision-making process of the birth, and to women who want to remain open to the full experience of the birth, however it unfolds. A sacred birth happens when a woman and her baby are treated as the most important people at the birth. How could we have forgotten this?

Sometimes the birth occurs quietly, with little fuss; sometimes the mother is as noisy as the experience is intense. In a sacred birth, whatever the mother's emotional expression, she is unrushed, and centered in her birthing power. The atmosphere is complete and timeless. When the baby is given time to unfurl slowly and the first moments of meeting between parents and child are undisturbed, something changes.

Marianne[4] taught me a beautiful approach to sacred midwifery at Helen's home birth some months ago. Marianne is a midwife in private practice; Helen, a human rights lawyer, was far from home — she's Irish. Marianne had supported Helen for hours, and I arrived later to assist at the birth. The labor was hard work; Helen spent some time in the bath and some time pacing. She leaned against the wall or against Marianne during surges. Then, finally, she squatted to give birth, leaning back against me after each surge. Her baby inched down the birth canal. Slowly the top of his head became visible, disappeared again and finally emerged, inch by inch, as Helen pushed and breathed and pushed again.

Paris was born onto a towel on the bathroom floor. He lay there, curled quietly, and covered in creamy vernix. Helen leaned back in exhaustion, and we waited. Marianne gently wiped Paris's mouth and sat back on her heels. He lay there, unmoving but still receiving oxygen through the pulsing umbilical cord. We waited and waited and it was difficult not to interrupt this moment. Finally, Helen leaned forward slowly, cooing softly. She touched him with her fingertip, he stirred, and she gently lifted him up onto her belly.

Helen was in a timeless state of being with her baby, and we were there with her. It was a numinous moment. There were no candles, no soft music playing, just the four of us in a warm and poky bathroom, sitting on the floor, surrounded by towels and birthing paraphernalia. And yet you could almost hear the universe singing. Paris is now eight months old and is so settled in his body and so strongly *present*.

Attending births wherein this sacred aspect is honoured gives us the time and space to sense a newborn's wisdom. If we slow down and pay real attention to our babies, by attuning ourselves to their rhythm, we gradually become aware of the meaning of their preverbal language, and life becomes more comfortable and welcoming for them. A baby can feel when we're fully focused on her, and she can feel the quality of our attention. She knows if she's held with love, knows if her parents feel confident and relaxed, knows how people around her are feeling. Most of all, she senses if we're responding to her with honesty. So if we're feeling ambivalent or overwhelmed, she will be okay with that if she senses that we're acknowledging what we're feeling.

Awakening to an awareness of the vulnerable, unharmed hearts of our babies, we can't help but take a bit more care with them. If we were to do so consistently, wouldn't it make a difference to our world?

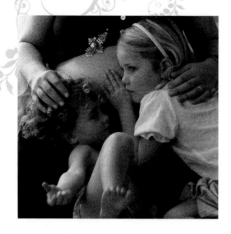

Talia and Amy chatting to Joel in Lindy's tummy.

Lindy's four births

Lindy gave birth four times. Her first baby was born by Caesarean section, and the three thereafter were natural births in a hospital setting. Lindy experienced life in its fullest expression during her births and her descriptions of them are true examples of the ability we have to experience ecstatic birth in actuality.

Birth is a spiritual initiation. Each birth is an initiation. We're so privileged as women. I was privileged to experience birth four times.

I fell in love with everybody in the room — the midwife, my partner Ronnie, the candles, everything. I was in a state of euphoria. I never had transition. I would get deeper and deeper into labor, into the breathing; the endorphins were so high — like the most potent meditation. There was total focus. By the fourth birth it was so intimate.

I have an interesting physiological thing: the baby's head never comes down, so I never have the feeling of the head on the cervix, just a feeling of opening, opening, like riding waves. The hard part for me is the pushing — it is hectic.

Birth is like a continuum, when we don't come to label or judge anything: small pain, huge pain, etcetera. Pain is just a physical sensation, and orgasm is a physical sensation; birth is a continuum of all of it. You can be in it and breathe in the most natural way, without having to use techniques. It's about being 100 percent present, into what is. This is why it makes sense that it's the most powerful spiritual experience you can have.

In so many religions it's believed that women don't need the ritualistic aspects to get closer to Source. So much of that is about birthing as a spiritual initiation. Can you step off the edge of the world? In labor, when you're really present, you come to the edge of all the things you know and you step into the darkness of the unknown. Can you do that? Can you just trust? Into the space that is so unknown—into the Void.

Spiritually, it feels like the Universe with nothing in it. It feels like the huge open space of nothingness. You don't exist anymore. At that point there's nobody in the room with you, no human being. You're not there. It's like death—the eternal space of nothingness. In that space, God or Spirit enters the room. That is the space where you go in birth.

Birth is the most spiritual experience, like gateways opening, like being not of this world, out of this world, a connection with the Void. Then there is such a different Presence in the room. Then, when I'm fully dilated, I feel like I want to go home, and then the work starts. For me the pushing is extremely hard work.

Talia's birth *was a twenty-seven-hour labor ending in Caesarean section, and I didn't even have pyjamas packed. It's amazing I had to have that experience. I was completely devoted to the idea of natural birth. I was fearless, confident. I was having it at home, and everything was going to be perfect. I think I had to accept the idea of not being in control.*

The birth was very traumatic for me, as I was terrified of hospitals. But I had to go through that to get a healthy baby and the realization that neither of us would have survived without the Caesarean—the acceptance that at a simple level I had never accepted allopathic medicine or surgery and I was too invested in that. I had to let go of being attached to natural birth.

I had a yoga teacher once who would demonstrate how it was as difficult for the supple student with the bendy back to hold her posture as it was for the inflexible student—they both had to come into balance. It's about what you have to work with to let go. This was an important lesson for me. The whole parenting story is one long journey of letting go. The first lesson of that is your birth: it's about letting go. Because I so wanted to let go into natural birth, I became over-invested in that, and so I had to let go of even that.

I hated the epidural. I felt like I was in one of those dreams you have at night where something terrible is happening and your legs won't move so you can't get where you need to go.

>

Talia was in trauma after the Caesarean and was taken away for forty-five minutes. At the Caesarean Ronnie could see what was happening, and he thought it wouldn't be traumatic—he had seen many births with farm animals before; but it was horrendously violent, and Talia was ripped out of my womb. I just saw this little girl with bangs, and she then was taken away. When she was brought back she looked deeply into my eyes first, and then into Ronnie's.

In Grade Five, Talia had to talk about something meaningful in her life to her class, and she told the story of her birth to her class as I had related it to her. But when she got to the part of looking into our eyes after birth, some visceral memory was stirred and she just started crying. It was a gift for her as a young child to return to her own birth.

I have experienced medical stuff, home birth and labor and epidurals and a Caesarean section—to have all that! The trauma of the birth didn't affect my bonding with Talia at all. She was ever more precious because of that trauma.

Amy's birth was what it was for me because of the first birth. I was told I couldn't have her naturally. Then I went to see the obstetrician, Justus Hofmeyer,[5] and he told me that in the United States women have a 75 percent chance of natural delivery after a Caesarean birth. Susan[6] was prepared to be my midwife, and in case of scar rupture, Amy was born at the natural birth unit at the Mary Mount Hospital. But it felt like I had three home births because of the way they were done. By the fourth birth, my kids didn't even know we had left home.

Amy's birth was relatively quick. I was more and more spiritually involved with each one. The spiritual experience got deeper with each birth, took me closer to Source each time in the labor. They didn't get easier, though. Joel's birth was harder than Amy's birth, and Jaden was in a posterior position—his birth was fast and violent and quick. He says, "I came like an arrow into this world." He was like a missile.

With Amy, we didn't know what would happen. Because she was the first birth after the Caesarean, Sue said, "We're not pushing for more than half an hour." After twenty-five minutes Sue gave me an episiotomy, and Amy just slipped into the world. She wasn't stressed, she was pink and beautiful. I was always in the water for my labors, but never birthed my babies in the water.

Amy's birth was thrilling, a thousand times more so because none of us expected it. In the first birth I was so invested in it being natural, and it didn't happen. That was preparation for parenting; not to be attached to anything, not even to a good thing, to good values.

With the second birth there was such a big difference: Ronnie, Sue, and I all went in open to anything. We weren't attached to the outcome—we knew it could end with a Caesarean; I even had a bag packed. So it could be what it could be. So we were in process. We were there for what was to be.

She came through beautifully. It was like being on the highest mountain, like walking on air. As soon as the baby was out, I put my boots on and we went home. Straight to my own bed. Coming home to Talia, it felt like a miracle. I think that's it: every birth is a miracle—not to take anything for granted.

Joel's birth: *An amazing thing is that Ronnie got Joel out. Ronnie was hugely involved in all the births, and he got Joel out of my body by psyching me with eye contact and strong support. I experienced spiritual stuff very hugely in that birth. Joel is a deeply energetically connected child. The Presence in the room was so spiritual that when I had to push him out I didn't know how to come into the physical act of pushing with my body. I felt that I couldn't come from that to this. That place I went to was so out there—the experience of coming back, from the ether into the most primal earth activity that you can imagine….*

Ronnie saw my power going, and he stood across the bed, firmly held my hands and my eyes, and he psyched me into getting my baby out. The people in the room are so critically important. Ronnie was perfect for that—he was so connected.

With birth and with art—going deeply into the unconscious, we need support. As an art facilitator, I hold a sacred space for my students for their art process; alone, it would be too scary for them to go there. Someone has to hold the earth space. Ronnie had to hold the earth space to bring Joel in.

Jaden's birth: *At half-past twelve at night, I phoned Sue and then my mum, who came to sleep in our bed. We went to Vincent Palotti Hospital. It was a radically quick, volcanic birth. Even though it was still so ecstatic—more so even, because the sensations were more intense.*

By six thirty that morning we were back home in bed with our baby. The children came into the room, and we were there in bed. He looked into each one of their eyes for a long time. I just knew that he'd come to meet them as much as he'd come to meet us; that there was a contract.

If you can just not judge birth, just experience it as it is, with no labeling or judgment. I've never been able to describe the experience of labor as pain. I know what pain is. Birth is a very strong sensation—to be able to experience very strong sensations, you have to be able to be open to life's power and force. Birth is like thunder. It is all that it is. Amy's birth was like a gentle lagoon—beautiful soft rain outside, so gentle. Jaden's birth was like thunder and lightning.

I had a book with photos of Iyengar's pregnant daughter in different postures, which I found at yoga classes with my first pregnancy. On one page she says: "You do not have to do anything when you give birth. There is nothing to learn. There are no techniques. Be present, be open, be a gateway." For me that was so important.

Now I understand why I had to experience everything for Talia—you can't be attached to anything. Birth is all about letting go. Preparation is all about learning to let go. Art classes for letting go. Breathing for letting go. It is so much to do with trust."

Life force

> "There is a vitality, a life force, an energy, a quickening, that is
> translated through you into action, and because there is only one
> of you in all time, this expression is unique. And if you block it,
> it will never exist through any other medium and will be lost. "
>
> — *Martha Graham, American dancer, and choreographer* [7]

Our bodies have an energetic system—a structure of subtle energy conduits acting as a connection between the spiritual dimensions of ourselves and our physical, psychological and mental bodies. This system also has the potential to connect us ultimately to the entire, energetic interaction of the Universe.

Twenty years ago, I became aware of this energy moving through my body during meditation. I was living in Botswana and had no spiritual teacher at the time, so because I was quite interested in this new development and kind of excited by the "specialness" of it, I worked too fast with it and blew open some closed-down areas. I think this is rather like putting too much energy through an electrical circuit and blowing the circuit.

This resulted in a bed-ridden, six-month period of extreme tiredness, with medical advice ranging from antidepressants being the only solution, to one less-than-lovely physician who decided that even though I was HIV negative, it was probably some latent form of AIDS that was yet to reveal itself in tests!

Eventually, my aunt, who has "healing hands"—quite a novelty in those days—sorted out the problem by giving me one twenty-minute session of her sort-of-but-not-quite reiki. She has no idea what she did, but I think she gently closed the blown-open areas again so I wasn't leaking too much energy through them in an unsustainable fashion.

My understanding of this "chi" or subtle energy, is that it is the life force that vibrates through our bodies; it is our fundamental quality of being and becoming. It is also the pulse of the Universe, and of every material object. It is both the potential and the actuality of any change taking place in our bodies. As has been known to Eastern medical science for thousands of years, this energy, or chi, flows through energetic conduits in our bodies, much the same as blood flows through vessels and capillaries. The flow of energy ought to be an open system connected to the flow of energy around us; however, in the bodies in which most of us live, although the chi is still flowing through us (otherwise we'd be dead), it is largely flowing through a closed circuit, disconnected from the sea of energy in which it floats.

Humans' subtle energy systems have vortices aligned at different points along them called chakras, which have the potential to open and connect with the energy in the Universe on a deep level, and in relationship with other beings and the world on a more superficial level. If any chakra is particularly tightly closed, or blown open without being centered enough to handle the flow of subtle energy this creates, it is often expressed through physical ailments and psychological stress. Conversely, physical ailments and particularly psychological stress serve to close the chakras down. Any time we encounter situations in which we don't want to stay fully present because they are uncomfortable for us, we suppress the feelings there and in order to do so we close down the energy flow at the point of our bodies where we are experiencing the uncomfortable sensation, be it either physical or psychological pain.

An enlightened person has a fully open chakra system. While I am told it is quite possible to become instantly enlightened, it seems to me it would be unlikely to occur unless the individual were prepared for it and their body's energetic circuits were capable of receiving intensely high frequencies of energy in mega-blasts.

Someone once described a mystic as being a person who is swimming in the same stuff that a psychotic is drowning in. A friend and neighbor of mine had a theory that when individuals take mind-expanding drugs such as LSD or ayahuasca, it can be likened to being a rosebud and desperately wanting to be in full bloom before your time, and ripping the petals open to see what it looks like inside. Our subtle energy systems open best through attention and love, especially through becoming aware of and loving the traumas and difficult experiences that have closed them down in the first place. Learning to gradually stay open to every situation as we encounter it creates health and well-being.

Open chakras allow energy to flow freely and easily though our bodies. The connection between our individual energy system and the universal energy in which we exist happens at any point in our bodies where we fully open our chakras. Each chakra relates to a different part of the body and to different psychological expressions. The chakras illustrate the interdependence of our minds and our bodies.

In most subtle energy systems, there are traditionally seven main chakras and many minor ones acknowledged in the body. There are also more below the feet and above the head, the lower ones serving to ground the individual, the upper ones to create a sense of connection to the Universe.

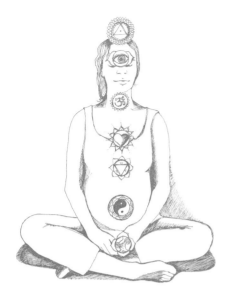

The seven primary chakras are energetically aligned along a central meridian in the body.

The seven main chakras

The seven main chakras in the body are found at specific points and relate to specific physiological and psychological states of well-being or disease.

The first chakra

Starting at the base of the spine, the first chakra is the root chakra. It symbolizes our consciousness taking individual human form on Earth, and the issues that it relates to are food, shelter and security. Our primal need and instinct for survival relate to this chakra. In our competitive society we often we get caught up in either spiritual or intellectual pursuits because somehow they seem grander and more elevating than basic physical needs. When we do this, the root chakra can close down. It's not so easy to enjoy life when we have no connection to the Earth, and when we are ungrounded it is very difficult to give birth. Since opening the root chakra is related to physical activity, staying healthy, getting lots of exercise, and working with the Earth—standing bare foot in soil, planting seeds, gardening, getting mucky sometimes—these all help to keep us grounded. Statistically, women who exercise regularly and are, therefore, more likely to be grounded, physical people—which means people with open root chakras – have easier labors.

The second chakra

The second or sacral chakra is referred to as the *tan tien* in Chinese culture or the *hara* in Japan. It is found about four centimeters (1.75 inches) below the navel and is connected to the sexual organs and to basic relationships with others, especially sexual and family relationships. The *tan tien* or *hara* is known as the center of gravity or the balancing point that martial artists, sumo wrestlers, and samurai warriors are grounded in. Years are spent simply developing an awareness of and strengthening the second chakra before martial artists can become masters.

A stronger *hara* relates to being less tired; it is a source of vital strength. In fact, it was this area in my body that I blew open with the excessive energy flow in my early thirties. Developing and strengthening this area creates a grounded and embodied access to vital energy. Breathing deeply into the belly at all times, rather than breathing in a shallow upper chest manner strengthens the *hara,* and centers and grounds us.

Shallow breathing is often indicative of a desire for perfection, which in itself is a sign of a rigid ego imprisoned in a "thinking" rather than "being" attitude. Strength in the *hara* can only be realized when we release the need to be seen as "someone" in other people's eyes. A strong *hara* is indicative of letting go of constantly striving for perfection at some point in the future. It requires simply recognizing that we are absolutely perfect just the way we are. That kind of acceptance is a wonderful attitude to bring to a birth room; it allows our babies to feel that they are okay just the way they are, too.

I attended a birth sometime back where the mother was constantly organizing us, the caregivers, in order to try and create her perfect birth experience. We settled in for the long haul, knowing that the birth was unlikely to take place until she moved out of her head and into her lower body more fully. Twenty-four hours later, she was eventually given a Caesarean section because her baby hadn't even descended into the pelvis yet. It is possible that her fear of surrendering into the process of birth kept her second chakra closed, and as such this could have contracted her pelvis physically by keeping it slightly more rigid.

Giving birth is essentially a first and second chakra affair, although giving birth consciously requires that all the chakras, and specifically the heart chakra, be wide open. Women labor best when their spirituality is grounded and fully embodied—when they are aware of their spirituality in a very physical way. Many of the exercises in this book are useful for gently activating closed-down chakras. The purpose of this is not simply to create a pretty "aura". There is an interdependence between energetic, physiological, and psychological states of being. A chakra that is open and clear has a significant relationship with the psychological state of responding to life occurrences rather than resisting and fighting them. This type of psychological health relates strongly to women who labor easily, whose cervixes melt open like butter, and who flow with the upheavals of life with a newborn. This doesn't mean that life and labor are perfect for women with healthy energetic systems. However, the buffeting becomes easier to weather when there is less resistance. Dance, such as belly dancing or trance dancing, can help to open the second chakra. Teenagers often play music with a heavy bass beat because the hormones of testosterone and estrogen overwhelming them have activated their second chakras and the bass beat resonates with open root and sacral chakras

Lisha kept her lower chakras open in labor. She speaks about the experience of letting go in labor as compared to previous contracted birth experiences as follows:

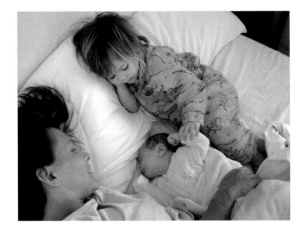

Lisha was so attuned to her body she could physically feel her cervix opening during each surge.

Lisha's birth story

After giving birth naturally twice before, this third birth experience was the most fantastic gift for me. My first two births were completely medically led—I had to have forceps deliveries with episiotomies, and an epidural with my second child, after an eighteen-hour labor! Much trauma for both me and my two daughters. The birth of my son—this last experience—was unbelievably beautiful! The labor progressed so quickly, which I believe was only due to the fact that I was totally relaxed through each contraction and the rests in between. I would not have been able to have been this relaxed without my birth companion continuously bringing me back to a state of absolute relaxation, enabling me to visualize the opening of my birth passage and the progress of the birth that each contraction brought. I could literally feel the baby moving down with each breath.

>

I can honestly confirm—having had the past two experiences that I've had—that tension prolongs labor and increases pain, whereas relaxation has the direct (extreme) opposite effect! The benefits of having such a birth have been amazing for both me and my baby. He is so much more relaxed and content compared to the first few weeks with my first two. (One might say this is because I have more experience this time around—I definitely say it's due to the peaceful birth experience we had!) The first time I heard him cry was when he was given the vitamin K injection.

My recovery was incredibly quick. Not having had to recover from stitches and the after-effects of an epidural, twelve hours after delivery I literally felt as though I'd never given birth! My advice to moms-to-be is to trust your body and know that the only control you have is to relax and hand your body over to the process!

The third chakra

The third chakra is centred in the solar plexus. It is the chakra that relates to personal recognition and power. Its elemental energy is fire, and opening it is motivated by a desire to develop an identity in the world. We are so often afraid of our power. We have very real knowledge hidden deep in our DNA, in our "collective unconscious", in the genes we inherited from our ancestors, that give us the ability to hurt ourselves and others through misusing our power. We all have access to both male and female power, but they take different forms.

We misuse female power by manipulating others in secretive, devious ways, and we misuse male power by killing, raping, and behaving destructively. When we are afraid of our power we close down our third chakras. Then, because they are weak and atrophied, we must cross our arms over our solar plexus to protect them from the world at large. Interestingly, in the Hindu chakra system, the presiding deity of this chakra, Bramha Rudra, represents the power of destruction.

Birth is one of the most empowering acts we ever participate in. It doesn't threaten other people, but moving into birth with a very real sense of our own power changes the experience. Women I know who are comfortable in their power have no problem asking for their needs to be met. Usually they don't even need to ask. Personal power is an attractive attribute; we all fall over ourselves trying to befriend people who are comfortably open in their third chakras.

Janneke was working with her unborn child last week. She is nine months pregnant and is someone I admire for having a clear, strong solar plexus. Yet that was just the area she chose to strengthen even more for the birth. She worked with golden yellows—the color of the solar plexus chakra—which protected her and made her feel strong. The feeling related to these colors was one of self-love, of being held as if someone else was crossing their arms over her solar plexus and keeping her safe. Her unborn child gave her affirmations to say about how beautiful and strong she is. There was a strong sense of non-judgment and trust throughout the session.

The fourth chakra

The fourth chakra is the heart chakra. It is the center point of the seven chakras, halfway between the three lower, more physical chakras and the upper, more ethereal and intellectual chakras. It is the seat of love, faith, devotion, and compassion.

In his book *A Path with Heart*, Jack Kornfield advises us: "In undertaking a spiritual life, what matters is simple: *We must make certain that our path is connected with our heart.*[8]" Even if all the other chakras are closed down, an open heart is the biggest, most beautiful thing. It's the chakra that babies relate to best; it's the one they're really good at cracking open. So even if yours is closed, a baby can open it right up. Opening chakras can hurt somewhat, because everything that keeps them closed comes to the surface for recognition before it is released. When our hearts are closed it is always because of some previous pain.

In *Shambhala, The Sacred Path of the Warrior,* Chogyam Trungpa[9] describes the tender heart of a spiritual warrior thus: "If you search for the awakened heart, if you put your hand through your rib cage and feel for it, there is nothing there but tenderness. You feel sore and soft, and if you open your eyes to the rest of the world, you feel tremendous sadness…. It is the pure, raw heart. Even if a mosquito lands on it, you feel so touched…. It is this tender heart that has the power to heal the world." And it is this tender heart that babies awaken within us. When I asked about love I was told by my spiritual guide: "Love is the greatest gift you will ever receive. It is the pearl beyond price. You only get to it by opening to your own pain and suffering. Hold this love in the midst of life, and then you realize that you are held at *all* times. That is all you need to know, but know it with every atom of your being."

Meditating, especially on loving kindness, is one of the most wonderful ways to work with gently opening the heart chakra.

The fifth chakra

The fifth chakra is the throat chakra. This is where we find our true sound. Each person has their own unique note that they have chosen to play. It is simply a matter of *playing* with it. Harmonic resonance is helped enormously by using sound and allowing the sound that is expressed through our throat to arise from a resonating chamber in our chest and belly. A clear and energized throat chakra adds profound beauty and power to our voices. The fifth chakra is related to the vastness of space; contentment and serenity arise here. A clear and open throat chakra motivates us to search for pure knowledge with clarity of awareness.

I attended a birth about a year ago, where the birthing woman had the power of an Amazon, and a loud voice. The entire neighbourhood knew she was in labor. However there was a long time at the end of labor when she was resisting the experience, so she would bellow "Nooo!" through each surge. Eventually she agreed to try changing the sound to a "yes." With some coaxing, she whispered "yes" during a surge. Although she never managed to bellow and truly affirm this "yes" with all of her being, actually saying "yes" instead of "no" changed something in the labor, so that very shortly after changing her birth mantra she moved from the work of cervical opening to that of pushing her baby out into the world.

The sixth chakra

The sixth chakra is located in the area of the third eye. Apparently, it is more or less where the pineal gland is found inside the head, which is the point where a horizontal line from between the eyebrows intersects with a perpendicular line from the crown chakra or anterior fontanel. This chakra resonates with the word "Aum," which symbolizes light. The sixth chakra represents austerity, clairvoyance, intuition, heightened mental faculties, and a state of self-realization. An open sixth chakra signifies an experience of life as being beyond time, space, and duality.

When we are working with the unborn child, they are always communicating with us from a place where they are beyond duality, judgment, time, and space. This brings a quality of wisdom into the communication that is quite astounding sometimes. Monica was given a gift from her unborn child of feeling joy and a connection with God. She perceived this as "a glow through my eyes and head, breathing it in there. It's like a sense of being connected, at one with myself, with Paul, with the Universe. A harmonizing, in synchrony with life." Her baby was helping her to open her sixth chakra.

The seventh chakra

The seventh chakra is located four centimeters (1.75 inches) above the point on our crowns where, as babies, we had the open soft spot of the anterior fontanel. It is a point that belongs both to the body and to the subtle energy beyond the body. This is the place where the primordial pulse of the Universe is experienced. It is a point of union with pure consciousness, without being disturbed by pleasure or pain, admiration or humiliation. Knowledge, the knower, and the known all become one. When the present Dalai Lama was recognized as a reincarnation of the previous Dalai Lama, he was three years old. He was allowed to remain with his parents until the age of five, before being taken to Lhasa as a tiny monk to be schooled and mentored for his position. Apparently, the most important instruction his parents were given for those two years was to never touch the top of his head, so as not to disturb his crown chakra and his point of union with pure consciousness.

In order to relate to the world at all we have to have some chakras at least partially open. As our chakras open, the universal energy of which we are a part—and in which we float like waves in the sea—can also flow more freely through us, so instead of being a closed system and holding tightly to an identity of a separate self, we begin to awaken to an experience of interdependence with all things. We are much like waves in the ocean: made of the same stuff but having an individual identity. Usually we see ourselves as the wave and not the ocean, and in creating such a separate sense of self we sever our connection to the ocean to which we belong and back into which we will eventually dissolve again. An enlightened being is one who has no boundaries whatsoever, who knows that their wave is only an expression of the ocean.

An open chakra creates a communication of energy between individuals and the outside world. We think we want to remain open and feel connected to the world at large. However, if someone sends us mean and hateful feelings they catch our energetic system at a point where it is open enough to receive the sensations. Because we don't like that, we either hurl these back instantaneously or shut down our chakra system to avoid the discomfort it creates, neither of which is a healthy solution to the attack. A person with a fully open chakra system has nowhere for such hooks to attach themselves, and therefore the nasty, spiteful energy simply slips right through them without ruffling or disturbing their peace of mind. They do this by simply experiencing the attack and feeling the sensations that it creates without attaching to whether this is a good or bad experience and without resistance to it. Someone this enlightened would stay non-judgmental in the face of the attack.

The enlightened person doesn't do this by shutting off their feeling and judgment, but by being so open to the universal energy flow that they have moved beyond the duality of good and bad and can see and understand the core wisdom and love that lies beneath the pain and suffering that causes us lesser mortals to hurt one another. When there is no resistance to a psychological attack, the person sending the hurt or hate then feels accepted enough that they no longer experience their own pain so intensely, which alleviates and releases some of their projections. And when we open to the surrounding energy on a deep level we perceive this sea of consciousness as profound, uninterrupted, unconditional love.

Transformation

The experience of opening the heart creates a quality of compassion and benevolence to flow through us. It sounds wonderful. It is wonderful. However, our separate selves can be uneasy in the presence of love which doesn't require us to behave in any particular way to win it, love that is utterly non-judgmental. We become uneasy because dissolving into it releases all our boundaries and diminishes our egoic sense of identity, the sense of "this is me." The "ego" being referred to here is our sense of having a separate self, an "I" with content. It does not refer to our sense of "ego" as "self worth."

We no longer have a reason for separate existence in the face of this love. It is so all-consuming that our separate sense of self burns up and withers away in its presence. And of course we don't like the idea of annihilation at all, we run from that faster than we run from wars, destruction and torment. Even though absolute annihilation is an entirely false presumption, we fear this destruction and the ego rightly persuades us that dissolving our boundaries will mean that there will be nothing left of "me."

Falling in love

Mostly we are not ready to face separate-self destruction. However, every fiber of our being still yearns for the connection with this unconditional love because we remember being part of it before we took on physical form and when we were in the womb. Often we choose to experience a reduced and more manageable form of this love through relationships, which is why we love the idea of falling in love.

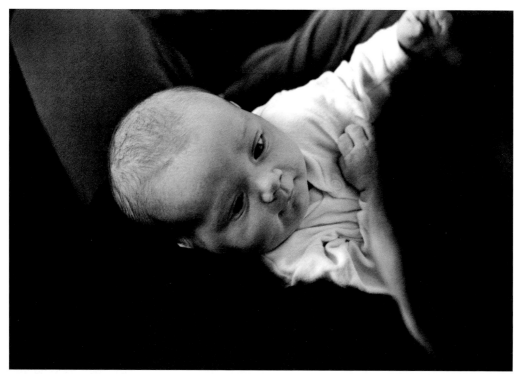

Klara gazing at her obviously gorgeous mother.

Because experiencing a sense of unconditional oceanic love is scary, we would prefer to cling to an idea of an individualized love, wherein someone will love us for being adorable and worthy. This is easier to accept than love that is available to us whether we deserve it or not. Many of us expect falling in love to be a positive or blissful state, but because we only open our heart chakra fully to the person with whom we have fallen in love (albeit with some fallout spilling beyond that person to make the world seem a happier, more glowing place and the people around us friendlier and more loving), it always creates pain and suffering for us when we become disconnected from our lover by either physical or psychological distance.

Not only do we long to be adored by a new lover, we also want to be adorable. The more extra-ordinarily perfect we can project ourselves to be and the more we are perceived as perfect and extraordinary by our loved one, the more we feel we are worthy and lovable inside ourselves, which of course comes with the downside that this illusion is entirely unsustainable.

35

Unconditional love

Babies and young children live in a world of unconditional love. We can pick our noses and they love us. Our farts and burps might even delight them. We are gorgeous in our lumpy hips, frumpy blouses, and milk-stained tracksuits. Our greasy hair and zits are not blemishes in the eyes of our babes. We can be exhausted and still they love us. We can be stressed and anxious and overwhelmed, and they cry for us in an attempt to bear our pain.

It is very easy to fall in love with tiny babies. They don't judge us; they simply love us because we are there. They love everything that is there, even though they already love humans more than other things, and they have a particular connection to their parents. And because they don't have barriers and defenses set up, we automatically diminish our barriers to come into some form of harmony and balance with them. In doing so we become more vulnerable, but we also love more intensely. We often allow our hearts to open more freely for our babies than for the other significant people in our lives, because they are less likely to hurt us if we do so.

Although painful experiences in the womb, birth trauma, or experiences of being unsupported in early life can diminish their open-heartedness, babies are often still bathed in what looks like pure bliss. Almost every parent can remember at some stage falling in love with their babies—falling into their unfathomable eyes. They gaze at us with soft intensity and because they have nowhere to go, nothing else to do, no one in particular to emulate, they meet us with full attention. This is unconditional love made palpable and packaged for individual consumption.

OPENING UP TO BIRTH

Chapter Two

> Giving birth in ecstasy: This is our birthright and our body's intent. Mother Nature, in her wisdom, prescribes birthing hormones that take us outside our usual state, so that we can be transformed on every level as we enter motherhood.
>
> — *Dr. Sarah J. Buckley, Australian MD* [10]

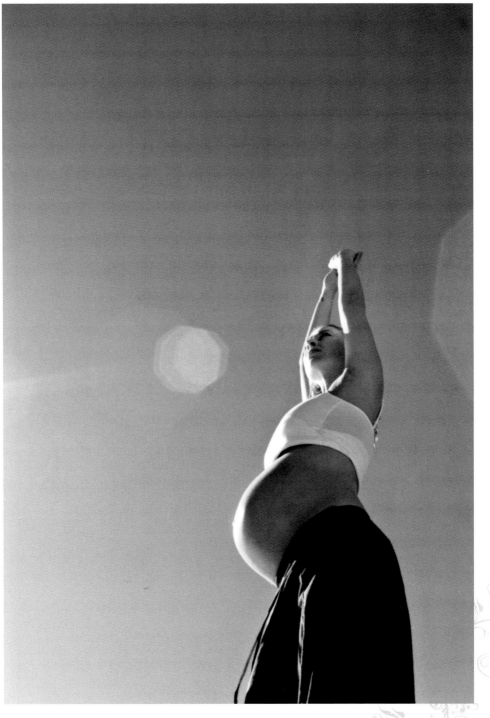

Mythological awareness of birth

" All religions and mythologies have creation myths. These myths can be quite fantastic according to the imagination of the people who created them and the environment in which those people lived. The gods in their mythical world have always closely mirrored the culture of the group that worships them. Thus, creation myths and birth rituals have always existed and have provided a meaningful conception of the origins of life. "

— *Phyllis Blakemore, Author*[11]

Birth has strong archetypal associations in every person's psyche. The more we minimize the significance of birth and escape its intensity, the more trivial it becomes in the collective consciousness, and the more we deprive our lives of meaningful experiences.

This morning the most beautiful woman, who had spent many long hours preparing for natural birth, required a Caesarean section for fetal distress, which happened after her obstetrician insisted on an induction for non-medical reasons. When I heard this, I needed to get out for a walk. So now I'm sitting at the edge of the sea on a long, raised rock on a promontory surrounded by waves, cormorants, and a gentle salty breeze. It's a beautiful day. Unrushed, the waves roll in, followed endlessly by others. The tide is coming in and is seeping slowly up to the base of my rock.

The tide rolls in faster now as I surrender to the impressions the Caesarean section has made on me. One more woman who longed to experience the beauty of birth and was robbed of it. One more baby deprived of a first impression of its world as a supportive and loving place. Control seems an ugly word to me today. In this wild place my heart is saddened for the baby who didn't experience the awesome nature of her birth. My heart cries out in pain for our world where we so casually strip life of meaning, strip birth of meaning.

Sometimes, women do not understand why they feel let down and saddened by their Caesarean births. Relatives and friends and the medical establishment all assure them that they really are fine, their baby is well, and they are misguided to believe that it would have been better any other way. Yet, often the feeling persists; it can last for years. Aldous Huxley wrote a book in the sixties called The Doors of Perception, describing the attempts he and his colleagues were making to "expand their perceptual horizons" with psychedelics. No matter the dubious means they used to get there, I've always liked the phrase and am particularly drawn to the concept when faced with society's view of birth as a medical non-event.

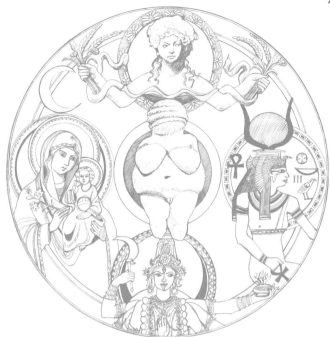

Birth archetypes. Centre: Venus of Willendorf, symbol of fertility.
Clockwise from left: Mother Mary, symbol of nurturing; Demeter, goddess of the harvest
and mother of Persephone; Egyptian goddess Hathor, symbol of female benevolence;
Kali, Hindu goddess of birth, creation, and destruction.

In many private hospitals these days, labor and birth are seen as fairly unnecessary. A nicely scheduled Caesarean will replace it effectively. The task of birth has been minimized and undervalued, like some unwanted and unused supermarket item that has passed its sell-by date. This is especially so when compared to the alternative of a scheduled Caesarean, which is so much more brightly packaged with marketing jingles such as "Save the beaver, have a Caesar." Mothering is just as undervalued. We sometimes view mothering as routine drudgery and a small and insignificant task—not a career at all, really. Yet birth has a mythological, symbolic, and archetypal force, which is associated with its feminine mystique and power. If we are to understand birth at all from a deeper level of reality, and if we are to discover its true worth, we must attend to its mythology and its mystery.

Honoring these archetypes can change our perceptions on a deeper level. Mothering archetypes are nurturing, life giving, unconditionally loving. Examples of them are Mother Mary in the West, Kwan Yin, goddess of compassion in the East, and Hathor in Ancient Egyptian mythological lore. These mother figures have a gentle power and a motherly sense of caring, but they lack the strength and creativity of birthing archetypes.

The primal birthing archetype is that of the Great Mother, of Mother Earth herself. Hesiod, a Greek poet from 700 B.C. states that Gaia, the Earth Mother, is the "oldest of divinities." In other words, she is the first, or primal, archetype. She gave birth to the gods. She is powerful as well as loving and supportive. She is destructive as well as creative. She is down to… earth!

The forces of nature belonging to our Earth Mother may be wrathful and powerful at times, and birth archetypes are often tightly interwoven with death in many cultures. The Indian goddess Kali, for instance, is both creator and destroyer, the bringer of life and death An archetypal Earth Mother is associated with instinctual actions, tenderness, protective-ness and with the expression of emotions.

When we give birth we are born as archetypal Mothers. Fearing birth, running away from it, reducing it to a procedure, is destructive to the power of women, to the power of the Mother archetype. We can recover it, but it is much harder than claiming it when it need not be learned—at the moment of giving birth.

The Birthing Mother archetype is close to the God archetype: God is creative, com-passionate, protective, all knowing, and is able to create order in the chaos. The birthing mother is creative: she births a human, she is compassionate and nurturing, she cares for her infant, and she is protective—the image of a lioness protecting her cubs is a pow-erful maternal archetype. Other animals traditionally symbolic of the Mother are bears and cows, while images of water, lakes, rivers, and the moon also express our concept of female energy.

Rachel Mendelson, mother of three home-birthed children, one of whom was born unassisted, has a deep trust in her own intuitive mothering abilities. These arise in part from her recognition of the meaning and symbolism of the mother archetype. She describes her sense of the Mother as "all-knowing, in the sense of having direct access to her feminine intuition, which understands hidden wisdom, and she is able to make sense of chaos and bring order and creativity into places of chaos. She is linked to the God archetype through the story of Adam and Eve. When children leave home (and mainly leave their mother), they are mythologically connected with being kicked out of the Garden of Eden, where Adam and Eve lived happily and naively while all their needs were met, and no problem and con-flict existed.

"We have many myths associated with leaving home and finding our way in the world— of leaving our mothers behind. In our Western world in all the powerful myths, the mother is absent. She is absent because she is so powerful. If the mother is there, there is no problem, no conflict. In order to become whole, it is necessary to leave the mother behind, for the hero or heroine to grow and do things by themselves and for themselves—to conquer fear, to be creative, courageous, to go on a quest to discover, to gain independence and to survive."[12]

Hansel and Gretel is a story of venturing out into the world, and the witch also represents the image of "bad mothering"—of being eaten up and consumed by the mother figure. The "bad mother" is a symbol of possessiveness, resulting in our inability to develop as individuals. I don't know much about The Iliad and The Odyssey, but I do know it wouldn't have been the same if Ulysses had never left home at all and his mum was still making him sandwiches for breakfast.

Many, if not most, mythological heroes are magically conceived or born. They are often placed in baskets, mangers, or seashells after birth. They are often set out on bodies of water to grow up alone without their mothers. Benig Mauger writes that "childbirth is an initiatory and transformative rite that evokes the archetype of the wounded mother."[13] It brings up all the unhealed mothering aspects of ourselves. She explores birth as an archetypal event of transformation, and pregnancy, childbirth, and being born as an initiation.

When we see birth as an archetypal event, it has significant psychological implications for our newborns. We then honor birth in a different way; we understand its ritualistic significance, its meaning in our lives. How we birth affects how we live. Interdependence is a quality that has long been overlooked and disregarded as insignificant in today's world.

Looking for interdependence brings a recognition that patterns of behavior do seem to repeat themselves, and they do often begin at birth. I have worked with a man who discovered that deep in his psyche, leaping out unbidden in a session, lay a strong correlation linking a Caesarean birth and isolation in an incubator with the same feeling when his father left for good when he was just two and a half, when he was sent to boarding school at age seven, and when his wife rejected him when she was pregnant. Life events that have a tremendous impact on us influence how we interact with the world later. One individual may hold onto significant trauma from her birth, while another who experiences a very similar birth pattern, may not register it as a trauma at all, but instead may hold onto a hurtful comment her mother made when she was three years old. The issues we do not release easily are those that create negative patterns of behavior in later life.

It is not essential that we recognize all our patterns and where they derive, but acknowledgement of the patterns allows us to recognize the holographic, multi-layered tapestry that is our life. The deeper meaning, the archetypal patterns, the interdependence, the psychological dramas, and the crude physical experiences each add a richness to the weaving that can look hollow and meaningless if we simply consider one layer at a time.

Miriam speaks of feeling connected to all women throughout time in her labor. Each surge drew her inward to a place where her awareness focused on the innumerable women who had been in this place before her. This knowing brought with it a sense of familiarity, of well-trodden ground. The images arising in her mind eased her labor by creating a sense of trust, because they connected her with the archetype of the birthing woman who knows it all in her bones.

Moving beyond fear

> " It may be worth considering that ultimate satisfaction with the experience of giving birth may not be related to lack of pain. "
>
> — *Dr. Sarah J. Buckley, Australian MD*[14]

Long ago I came across a book called *Love is Letting Go of Fear*.[15] It claimed that love and fear were opposing forces on one continuum, rather like hot and cold, or light and dark. Fear has been a strong presence in birthing rooms over the last two millennia, born out of a high mortality rate and a disregard for the birthing woman's need for support and love during labor. This fear impacts on how labor progresses and on our newborn's ability to trust in life.

Dr. Stanislav Grof and Dr. Arthur Janov have both worked extensively with primal memories and the bearing they have on our relationship with the world. Dr. Grof developed Holotropic Therapy for releasing birth traumas,[16] and Dr. Janov created the model of Primal Therapy, or the Primal Scream, for clearing the deeply-held negative patterns formed by birth memories.[17] We forget that how we were birthed is held deep in our unconscious mind and may influence on our emotional or mental well-being later in life. In order to move beyond our conditioning and to truly understand birthing realms we simply need to trust our bones. Those "I know it in my bones" bones. The most helpful thing we can learn intellectually for birth is that it's good to trust that knowing. In birth, there is nothing to do except let go. We have as little control over it as we do when we are a passenger on a roller-coaster. Some people love the thrill of a roller-coaster and, even though I'm not one of them, I'm guessing

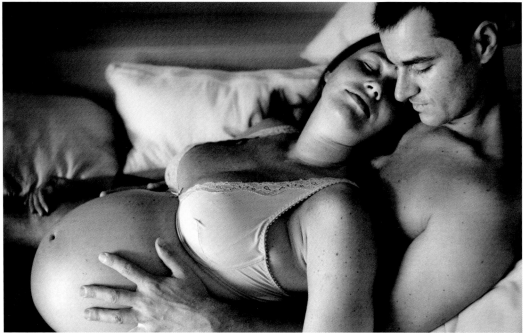

Surrendering into the experience of labor is the biggest factor in creating easy and natural births.

that they're the ones who relax and enjoy the ride. For me it's a fairly miserable experience because I wish I could check on the maintenance crew and don't really trust the machinery. If I were to take that attitude into a birth room, the chances are I would be creating a similarly miserable experience for myself there, too.

Birth is not governed by the conscious mind, which can keep control over its world. The birth computer lives in the limbic brain, alongside our intuitive knowings, and it is managed by the autonomic nervous system. Intellectual preparation doesn't even get through the door into that control room. Trusting our bodies is the best entry point, and "surrender" is the password. In English, we have no word for "surrender" that doesn't imply giving our power away. In Spanish, the word *"entrega"* describes surrender into the flow of life. It implies a voluptuous sense of harmony and delicious embracing of life, a letting go of our resistance. This is *"Wu Wei"* in Chinese, which means "the harmonization of one's personal will with the natural harmony and justice of Nature."[18] The English word implies that, we are meant to control life, harness it, make it bend to our needs and desires. This is bad news for birth. Control and resistance create fear and pain in birth, which lead to the need for more control and the buildup of more resistance and a huge desire to escape from the experience of the sensations. Hence, the popularity of Caesarean sections and epidurals.

Personally, I am built to keep control of my environment. I am well trained in the way of intercepting signals from others and adapting my behavior to conform to whatever will keep the status quo balanced and even. My life is a subtle play of keeping happy, keeping others happy, making sure everything is just so.

But labor just isn't proper and well behaved. It does have the potential to be calm, peaceful, and painless even, but to require it to be this way robs it of its power. Birth, like death, has no regard for social niceties. The bodies of birthing women shed mucus, blood, and shit with indelicate abandon. Our heads don't often approve of such behavior, but our bones know. Oh, they know, and they delight. They are so grateful for the opportunity to just be themselves.

Often when we give birth, we are young enough to still care very much about society's judgment of our behavior. "Bad" behavior still closes our hearts down into little balls of sadness at the expected parental disapproval, and we would do much to avoid that feeling. So it is up to us as women to change society's expectations of birth behavior, by understanding first for ourselves, that "good" behavior during birth entails trusting that our bodies know how to do this and that staying open to the sensations and emotions flooding through us during labor is part of the dance of birth. It puts us in touch with our "bone power." American poet Mary Oliver wrote a poem called *"Wild Geese,"* wherein she describes this knowing beautifully:

 ...You do not have to be good.
You do not have to walk on your knees
for a hundred miles through the desert, repenting.
You only have to let the soft animal of your body
love what it loves.

—*Mary Oliver, American poet* [19]

Trance rhythms

> Spirituality is like living water that springs up from the very depths of your own personal experience of faith. To drink from your own well is to reflect on your own unique encounter with the divine at the depth of your psyche.

—*Saint Bernard of Clairvaux, French abbot 1090-1153* [20]

There is a certain quality present at a birth that often reminds me of the San trance dances, which took place on the extremely remote farm I lived on in northwest Botswana in my twenties. This same quality was also palpable at sangoma tribal dances I attended. I think it arises from the sense of timelessness present at the dances.

I seldom participated actively in the dances. Sitting on an old log or a ratty piece of woven garden furniture, timelessness washing through me, I would be mesmerized by the rhythm created from the repetitive stamping of the dancer's ankle rattles and from their haunting chants, while immense dark skies and brilliant stars made a high-pitched universal hum in my ears. My memory of those nights invokes the feeling of winter cold biting at my neck, my shoulders, and at my behind through the gaps in the chairs, while the huge fire roasted my cheeks, my nose, and my hands. I was entranced by the feeling of simply settling into myself, this same rhythm and cadence of birth settles me, knowing that birth simply takes as long as it takes.

During undisturbed births, we fall into a trance like state toward the end of our labors. We can hear what is happening outside our bodies and answer questions, if need be, but the outside world seems far removed, and we are deeply sunk into that primal birthing space where we create our own sounds, our own world. All that concerns us at this time is the rhythm of the labor itself, the ebb and the flow of it, powerful surges gripping us and washing through us, then releasing us into restful phases of regeneration.

Trance is a universal phenomenon, and part of the power of birth derives from this unknown trance place. Much of our fear of birth may stem from an unwillingness to go into these dark and unknown places. Dance and the intimacy of being truly loved in labor create the necessary support for surrendering and letting go in birth. They can help us to welcome the experience and to gradually soften and open.

Support is a very necessary condition for most of us when we are entering into the trance-like space of our limbic brains—into that space where dreams are made. We must feel safe and we need to be comfortable in the knowledge that somebody out there is

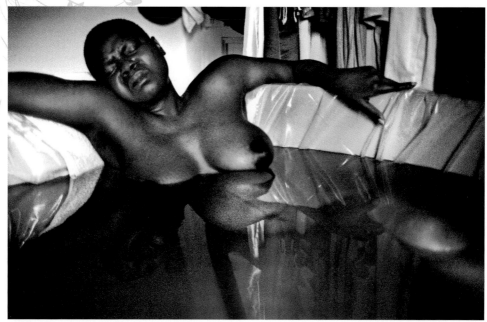

Women naturally move into a deeply internal trance like state in undisturbed labors.

looking after our physical well-being. Worry and anxiety interfere with entering any form of trance. Trance is an altered state of awareness that takes us into the shallows or depths of that sea beyond our everyday concept of reality.

Using visualization techniques to learn to become comfortable deep inside the self, and then using dance to lend a feeling of support, intimacy, and love to the process, we are more willing to enter the trance like state that is the natural domain of labor without resistance or fear. When we use deep relaxation to connect with our unborn children prior to our labors, we are often advised by our babies that remaining aware of their part in the work of labor is helpful, not only to us but to them as well. Labor can become a dance of connectedness us as birthing women, our partners, the energy in the room, our birthing babies, and every person who wanders in and out of the birth place.

However, because this concept of labor and birth is still uncommon and has long been forgotten by our collective consciousness, we need to prepare and train and relearn how to birth in a state of grace. We do this not only for ourselves but for our children—to help ease their way into this world. And also, ultimately, for the collective consciousness to relearn that if we birth free of trauma, we have the potential to live on this planet with less fear and less need to fight to protect our emotional well-being.

Good enough

" Water that is too pure has no fish. **"**

— *Ts'ai Ken T'an*

"Not good enough" has the strongest impact on labor, birth, and motherhood in our First World consciousness. The biggest drawback of our medical system is that we are labelled as "patients" during birth—patients whose bodies are not good enough to labor without help or interference.

There are symbolic messages in the machines, in staff attitudes, in obstetric tones and answers given to our questions that all imply that we're going to need all the help we can get because our birthing bodies are designed to malfunction. Given the lack of trust and fear around birth, it is hard for our bodies not to comply with these expectationst, and many of us find it almost a relief to hand our bodies over to the experts, thus reinforcing a sense of "not good enough" into our already wobbly self-esteems. Not trusting our own bodies, it becomes very difficult to trust that our babies can live and breathe and play in this world without an underlying dread that we or they may get it wrong with the direst of consequences.

My work with pregnant women who are connecting to their babies using integration therapy demonstrates that these wise babies understand that not only are circumstances perfect in the way they unfold but that they, too, are perfect at the deepest level. They hold abundant unconditional love for their parents and all beings because they also hold love for themselves. They are still beyond judgments created by the duality of good and bad.

At birth, babies apparently experience a sensation of being squashed into their bodies, which feel heavy, clumsy, fairly awkward, and very limiting. Simultaneously, their little bodies can also feel wondrous, new, and exciting, if they are met with love and acceptance and if they have endorphins and oxytocin in their system from their mother experiencing natural, fear-free labor.

It is in the early transition period after birth that babies in our First World culture often encounter the experience of 'not good enough'. If we as parents believe we are not good enough, we transmit it directly to our babies in the way we hold them and through the way we hold ourselves. Wanting to do things perfectly is a very clear expression of "not good enough."

A woman who was a tremendously successful interior designer in her previous pre-baby life, felt awkward and unsure in her first days of motherhood. She couldn't read baby signals, her baby felt alien and fragile and so very little, and she was used to being competent; in fact, her sense of who she was hinged in large part on being well thought of by her peers for career

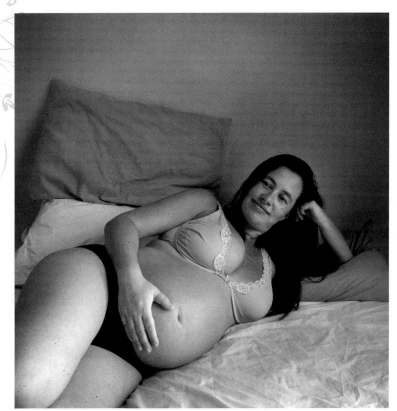

Petra's body is good enough. She has a comforting sense of being at ease with it, just the way it is.

competence and reliability. She was also witty, confident, and fun to be around socially. So on top of her awkward unsureness, she placed a determined expectation of herself as perfect mother—a mother who was quite assuredly "good." In her eyes, this translated as a reliable, happy, loving mother with a content and cuddly baby. One whiff of this expectation that he should be other than he was, that neither of them was quite good enough just the way they were, and her baby's tiny tummy contracted in a tight defensive ball of resistance and fear, leading to months of painful crying, accompanied by guilt, exhaustion, and postpartum depression, and for his mother, feelings of being overwhelmed and of losing control.

In our society, we don't have enough matriarchs reassuring us that we're okay. That it's okay to not get it right the first time, and it's okay to weep over our vulnerability at the awfulness of things and at being fairly rotten at this new job. "Good enough" is not a measure we are judged against. "Good enough" is simply taking responsibility for being who we are, preferably with a lot of people loving us along the way.

Opening and surrender

" In this life we cannot do great things. We can only do small things with great love. "

—*Mother Teresa, Nobel Peace Prize winner*

Having babies can create the opportunity to see the world in a new way. Actually, it's an old way. Babies can remind us to see the world through their eyes, in the way we used to interact with the world as babies ourselves—filled with innocence and openness, seeing the mountain through the window, hawks soaring, the citrus tree heavy with fruit and with life, each thing just as it is, as yet unclouded by hurry and worry and the stains of growing older, wiser, and more jaded. Our children can remind us adults to breathe into this world, but this time we do so with conscious, cognitive awareness. No longer victims of circumstance, we bring our experience and wisdom to each encounter. Slowing down and reopening childlike eyes, as adults we are more aware of the condition of being human, of our life as a process of change and as an intricate dance between the dark and the light.

There are opportunities for immense spiritual growth available to birthing women, which may not be present so easily at any other time. These opportunities exist more fundamentally for women than for men for a number of reasons.

Since we carry our babies inside our bodies for nine months, we are intimately connected to their energetic system, which is more open to the universal energy flow than ours. As adults, uncomfortable life situations have usually given us painful lessons in closing down and resisting the experience of being here. Unfortunately, refraining from immersing ourselves in the pain, grief, or rage we are afraid of experiencing, also denies us the opportunity to become fully engaged in the vitality and sparkle of our existence. Carrying an energy of new life within our wombs reminds us of the possibility of connecting to and absorbing our experiences in a more abundant manner.

As women, we have the opportunity to experience the intensity of childbirth in a powerfully physical way, while our male partners can only truly experience it emotionally. This intensity can be so overwhelming it can force us to surrender to the experience without avoidance. Often the only way our cervixes will dilate easily is by yielding fully to the power of birth, evoking a distant reminder of our potential to surrender our egos to life whenever we experience spiritual awakenings.

As women we are often left at home with our babies for long periods of time—in this day and age, usually on our own. It can be a lonely, even frightening time, one of inadequacy and unknowing, yet the softening and blossoming of our hearts at this time can be immense. The scent of our babies, their soft mewlings, utter dependency, and silky delicate skin tears at our hearts, floods us with endorphins, and we find we cannot resist the unconditional love they exude. Tiny babies don't judge us; they simply love us because we are there. They love everything that is there. Because they don't have barriers and defences set up, we automatically diminish our barriers to come into some form of harmony and balance with them. In doing so we become more vulnerable, but we also love more intensely. We often allow our hearts to open more freely for our babies than for the other significant people in our lives, because they are less likely to hurt us than adults, who are filled with judgments, expectations, and resistances.

For both women and men, the interval surrounding birth is a liminal phase in life. A liminal state represents a border zone between one stage of being and the next. This stage is characterized by ambiguity, openness, and indeterminacy. Our sense of identity dissolves to some extent, bringing about disorientation, but also opening the way to something new. Often when a new baby enters our lives, particularly if we haven't experienced being parents before, we are thrown into this state of uncertainty; we don't feel like new parents yet, we are still unsure, we have yet to get our bearings. This hesitation creates a window in our normally more rigid patterns of thinking and behavior.

The birth of a newborn is not only a new experience; it is also one where we feel unconditionally loved, sometimes for the very first time in our lives. This can create a safety net to surrender fully into the new experience without resistance. If we do so consciously and with an understanding of how and why we are doing so, we have the opportunity to remain more open as our babies grow, to actually transform ourselves through learning from our babies.

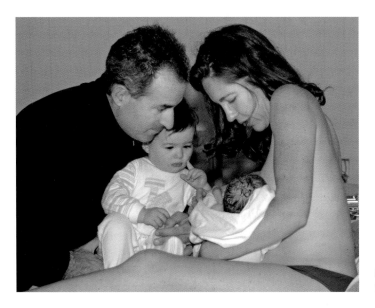

Darron, Gabriela,
Dru, and Christina.

Christina's second birth

Christina's cousin's baby had died at a home birth. So for Gabriela, Christina's first baby, she was under a lot of family pressure to have her baby in the hospital, and she did in fact, transfer to hospital during the labor.

Dru's birth was one that Christina described as: *"Phenomenal and quite the most amazing experience. I completed a Birth Transition course just prior to Dru's birth enabling me to be a doula for my own birth. A doulas works with both the father and mother, connecting them with the incoming soul over the whole pregnancy and birth, enabling the mother to have a conscious beautiful birth and the unborn child to have a much smoother transition into this world. This training totally changed my husband and my birthing experience and our connection with our child Dru prior to his arrival.*

We were taught to access a higher level of consciousness during birthing. One of the profound differences between Gabriela [our firstborn] and Dru's birth was that, at Dru's birth, I accessed a celestial birthing energy (pinkish in color). It was amazing. I felt like I had a genie's lamp. Anything I thought of, I could just mani- >

fest. I had powers I had never dreamed of, I could call on this energy to help with any moments of fear by just visualizing this pink light. My mom, who was meditating in her bedroom, four rooms away, said she could literally see sparkles of light coming down into the birthing room.

I had done a lot of clearing after Gabriela's birth because I didn't know how I was going to be able to get through the pain of the transition part of the labor again. I used EFT (Emotional Freedom Techniques) for clearing fear and anxiety prior to the birth, and during the birth for pain and discomfort. Each time I used it I had at least four pain-free surges.

The toning that Robyn put me onto, I didn't know if I could do. I never practiced it. I never heard anyone do it. Yet as soon as the surges started, I began to tone. It really helped. I found the toning, the EFT, and the angelic energy fantastic. I felt like there was so much angelic support. I used it to connect to Dru, and also each time I felt like things might be about to become a little tough. They never did, though.

The biggest difference for me in the two births was with Gabriela's birth I was taught how to relax, but in Dru's birth I decided not to be reactive to the surges. I would go into my cervix mentally—I'd join Dru there, be in my pelvis with him. We determined together how strong the surges would be, when they would come, and that I did not need many surges to reach full dilation. I did everything in consultation with Dru. I felt like we were a great team. When I was eight centimeters (3.5 inches) dilated, Sue [my midwife] suggested I get in the water. Then I was only having one surge every ten minutes or so. I didn't need many surges to get to full dilation. With each surge I went into the cervix and visualized it opening. Every surge was a different flower. It helps at times like these to have a sister who is a botanist! The last surge was a magnolia flower. They were my grandmother's favorite flowers—the grandmother after whom Gabriela is named. I felt she was letting me know that she was there.

My surges started at midnight. I wanted to give birth by 6 a.m., before my daughter woke. They started slowly. I was really calm and just toned. My husband called Sue when we thought I may be in proper labor, but I was unsure as things seemed so easy… By the time she arrived I was five centimeters (1.97 inches) dilated already. When I was in the water it all slowed down. Sue remembers me saying 'I'm not feeling anything.' I was in a space of immense power; I felt I could do anything. I had the ability to bring on a surge when there wasn't one, to tone and have no pain, to visualize my cervix opening and then, when Sue checked me, I was two centimeters (0.79 inches) *more dilated than half an hour before. The surges didn't get stronger after my waters broke. At the very end I had two strong surges, and there was marginal discomfort, but only for ten to twenty seconds. I said to Sue, 'Won't you just catch the baby?' She said 'What? You went from fully dilated to crowning in half a push!' He was born in the water. We kept the placenta attached for quite a while after the umbilical cord had stopped pulsating. I kept asking him if he was happy to have it cut. He said 'No' until he was ready.*

I used Dru's input the whole time. Every time Sue measured his heartbeat he was so relaxed. His heartbeat was variable but relaxed. We felt so connected through the whole process.

I was very present. I was so relaxed, I keep on talking to Sue as if birthing was no big deal. Toning dissipated any energy blockages, as did the EFT. Sue thought it was the perfect birth. It wasn't so quick that she felt rushed in any way. But it was so relaxed for her, too—six hours from the very first painless surge to holding Dru. They never got closer than three or four minutes apart, and they didn't last more than a minute. I was just bringing them on when I was ready.

The experience Robyn gave me with the unborn-child work, which we did early in the pregnancy, was very empowering. I saw him looking so much like he does now. He gave me strength and confidence to face the birth. I really needed that support. It was such a blessing that Robyn couldn't be my doula. I had to play that role myself. I had to empower myself. I felt like I was writing the biggest exam ever. I wondered if I could do it, without running to the hospital for an epidural. Afterward, I felt like I had finished university with an A grade.

Sue and Ciska, who attended Christina's birthing as midwives, added their comments to her birth story.

Sue: *"What stood out for me most at Christina's birth was how mentally she was completely in synch with every aspect of the birth. She could almost summon the surges. There was a crazy scenario between when she was eight centimeters (3.5 inches) and ten centimeters (3.94 inches) dilated. She was in the water and seemed a bit fed up because they were 'a bit far apart.' The next surge she leaned back and her baby's head was crowning; it was like she made this mental decision 'I want to meet my baby now'. She had none of the usual signs of feeling pressure, just the head crowning."*

>

Ciska: *What stood out for me was the healing that came from Dru's amazing birth. Healing of any trauma from her [Christina's] first birth, which was understandably fear-based. Since the birth of Gabriela, Christina has come into herself.*

Love makes birth easier. If women can put fear aside and really feel love—for themselves, their process, and their baby. There needs to be a feeling of well-being and of safety. Women need a strong belief that birth is natural and that they can do it.

On a practical note, women must get out of their heads and let go of being too controling. Christina was following the flow of her own process, rather than over-managing her birth.

Loving all of life – good and bad

> 'All love is the love of God' soul declares and plunges into the first kiss, into a glass of Shiraz, into saving the planet, into eating a bowl of steamed clams, into remodeling the kitchen.

—*John Tarrant, Zen Buddhist psychotherapist* [21]

Loving life and perfecting life are opposites on the life continuum. Loving life doesn't mean forcing or molding it into lovable form. Life is never going to be perfect, because even the perfect moments will change, and we often spend those moments anticipating this. In most of my perfect moments, I'm very soon distracted into fantasizing about them, thinking about what I should remember for later, or wondering about what I could add to the moment to make it even more perfect.

Loving life happens when we embrace life just as it is. Being exhausted or overwhelmed with a new baby can be recognized as simply a layer in a multitude of parenting experiences that create an interwoven whole of extreme richness and variety. Difficult experiences belong to life as much as previous partying till dawn may have done. Parenting includes within it feelings of frustration at not knowing baby language; warm, heart-melting connections; sore nipples; soft vulnerability. We can't embrace one of these feelings and reject the others. They belong together.

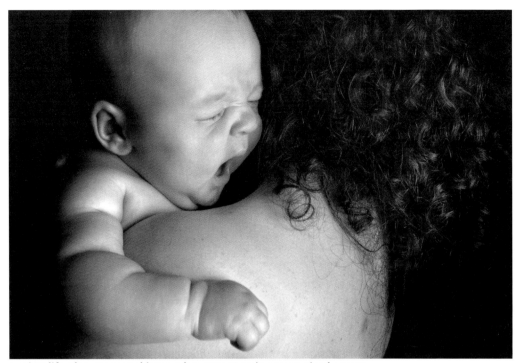

Loving life also means taking each moment as it comes, tired or not

Open acceptance of each moment doesn't exclude changing what needs to be changed. When we're exhausted, and it's eleven in the morning, we can sleep when our babies allow it, and we can arrange a support system of grannies, friends, and spouses when they won't. There is no such thing as embracing life and rejecting ourselves. Loving life includes flabby bellies, cellulite, postpartum pimples, and unwashed hair. It includes accepting those moments when we're horrid and nothing like the Earth Mother we're supposed to be. It also includes mourning what we've lost in terms of independence, freedom, and lack of responsibility. Breathing into all of this, noticing the dragonfly outside the window in the sunlight while delicious baby smells wash through our tiredness, is the surrendering into the "wow" of what can be termed loving life.

Harmonic resonance

" People say that what we're all seeking is a meaning for life... I think that what we're seeking is an experience of being alive, so that we actually feel the rapture of being alive. "

—Joseph Campbell, American mythology professor and writer[22]

When I was a schoolgirl I visited the National Art Gallery in Cape Town because enormous stone and bronze statues by Henry Moore had been flown out from the United States as a traveling exhibition. The curator of the gallery told us that the only way to really "see" the sculptures was to close our eyes and to touch the sculptures with our fingers as a blind person would. I "saw" the sculptures with my body, and they touched me back. It had such a profound effect on me that I spent the following four years studying art at university because I wanted to be able to touch people the way Henry Moore had touched me.

Last night I listened to Antonio Forcione, a Spanish guitarist, play inspiring solos in an auditorium with beautiful acoustics called the Whale Well (because it is strung with flying whale skeletons). Forcione's entire body listened to his music as he played. At the start of his playing, he seemed to be aware of his shoulder and of releasing it, so that the music flowed through his arms. His body responded subtly to the music—an opening of his chest, a bending of his head. He was feeling his way through the music with his fingers, and the rest of his body surrendered into this process and was an integral part of the music.

The movie *As it is in Heaven* was spectacularly popular for an art movie with subtitles. The theme of the movie centered around the characters finding their true sound through toning. Toning resonates through open chakras and allows us to recognize where they are closed. This has tremendous implications for use as a birthing tool. I read an article by Ingrid Bauer some years ago in *Midwifery Today*. It was entitled "Birth as sheer pleasure."[23] The author described her labor as being so wonderful, so physically exhilarating, that to describe it as "pain free" was akin to describing a gorgeous sunset as "ugly free." Watching the guitarist play his music last night, I remembered that Bauer had mentioned that she was a singer and had "toned" sounds throughout her labor. Toning creates a harmonic resonance in the body, wherein the subtle energy aligns the cells in a harmonic pattern of energy flow. (See Toning and Singing, page 131.)

This same resonance is created by aligning the senses, so that it becomes possible to hear music in the chest and heart areas, or throbbing through the belly and limbs in a rhythmic pulse, or to "see"' with the fingers, or to assign a color or texture to an emotion or

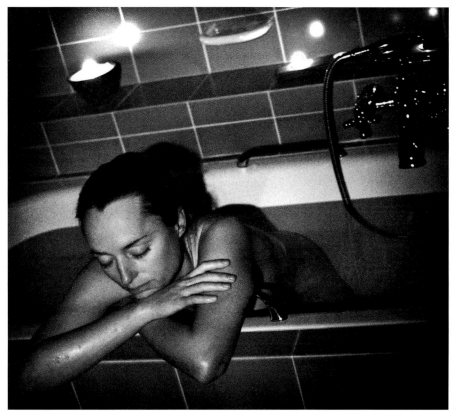

Surrendering into each moment as it arises creates an internal harmony in the body that helps the cervix to release into full dilation.

sound. When the senses are aligned enough to cross over and blend into one another we are in an energetically attuned place that is open and surrendered into the moment. It is a powerful place to be in for birth and for child rearing.

Harmonic resonance occurs when we are at peace with the events occurring around us. It is unusual in our world to settle into the present for more than brief moments of time, and even peak experiences may be interrupted by mind wanderings and imagining the retelling of the moment or how it would look through someone else's eyes. Falling fully into the moment, boundaries dissolve, creating a rhythmic cadence of merging into the universal ebb and flow of self and other. The present moment dissolves into timelessness, and the experience of unity is far greater than the sum of the parts creating it.

Moments of creative genius, of pure vitality, of really listening to someone, of intense sexuality, and of spiritual transcendence all bring us into resonance with our life force.[24] The unusual power of birth lies in our ability at this time to fully merge with our creativity, our vitality, our ability to listen, our sexuality, and our spirituality, simultaneously. Yet the only way to do so is through complete surrender into the intensity of the experience.

This same sense of harmonic resonance creates the quality of attention that helps babies to settle into their bodies after birth. Alexia and Mark had a difficult twenty-four-hour labor, ending in a Caesarean section. Although their baby, Klara, latched easily, she was physically sore from the birth. She cried when she was touched and became distressed when the many nurses picked her up and jiggled her. So Alexia and Mark asked to be disturbed as little as possible, darkened the room, and for twenty-four hours they lay quietly together with Klara in the hospital and simply gave her soft, focused attention—a feeling of being fully there for her. They came into harmonic resonance with themselves, with her, and with their surroundings, whereupon Klara relaxed, unwound, and settled into her body.

Birth hormones

66 A revolution will occur in our vision of violence when the birth process comes to be seen as a critical period in the development of the capacity to love. 99

—*Michel Odent, French endocrinologist* [25]

Undisturbed and fear-free births have an emotional impact on the babies we are birthing. It is not a myth that babies can smile at birth; they often do, if they are not shocked and emotionally withdrawn at birth.

Usually babies are born with the doctor or midwife making the decisions and directing the birth. Sometimes, the mother takes more responsibility for her body and decides how she would like the birth to take place. Occasionally, birth is left to follow its own natural course, and then, possibly, the baby has some control over how and when it will be born.

Dr. Michel Odent is a highly acclaimed endocrinologist and midwife, who maintains that women know intuitively how to give birth. Not only do we as women know how to birth instinctively, but Michel Odent believes that if we allow them to be so, our babies are actively involved in the birth process, too. They participate in the initiation of their own birth by stimulating the production of birthing hormones in their mothers. In doing so, they may also be training themselves to produce their own oxytocin. Oxytocin not only produces the ejaculatory reflexes of birth contractions, semen ejaculation, orgasm, and milk let-down but it is also associated with the feeling of love.

Dr. Odent maintains that our significant inability to love ourselves and others in our modern world may possibly be traced back to the time of birth and to the way we interfere with the production of the love hormone oxytocin with medical interventions. The Dalai Lama, when asked about how we should deal with the problem in our society of low self-esteem, and lack of self-love, held his chin, frowned slightly, and proclaimed that he believed this particular malady must be "rare, very rare" and that it was unheard of in Tibet.

Dr. Odent studies the impact hormones play in our perception of events, and he recognizes the central role of hormones in the childbirth process. He advises that the birth should occur in a quiet, safe environment with as little intervention and interference from the birth assistants as possible. Our most basic needs in labor are for privacy and intimacy, which help us feel safe and secure enough to give birth without fear. This allows us to trust our environment enough so that we can slip into the limbic part of our brains and let the neocortex, or rational part of the brain—step aside for a while. We then have the potential to birth in the way that other mammals do—quietly and fearlessly.

Our rational, intellectual neocortex interferes with the process of birth and with the production of birthing hormones. In order to birth as naturally as possible, we need to allow for the birth hormones, oxytocin and endorphins, to be produced without the interruption of adrenaline, the fight/flight hormone that most of us produce at low levels all the time, and then crank up to fever pitch during times of excitement and fear like birth. The most important thing for easy birthing, Odent suggests, is for the mother to disengage her neocortex during birth, and reengage her primal, intuitive brain instead.

Apparently, stimulating the neocortex through being efficient, intellectual, and organized causes the hypothalamus to produce adrenaline under the intense conditions of labor and birth. This in turn creates the fight/flight syndrome; and the more fear we produce in labor, the more the pain/fear cycle intensifies. This is true whether the threat producing the adrenaline is a current physical reality or the unconscious memory or expectation of trauma. Questions like, "How are you doing, dearie?" or too many directions from the birth team keep our neocortexes actively processing information, and thus can send a constant stream of adrenaline through our bodies. High levels of adrenaline during labor increase the duration of labor and can cause distress to our babies and slow their heart rate patterns down.

Immediately prior to the undisturbed birth of our babies, we will naturally produce a strong cocktail of both adrenaline and oxytocin simultaneously. This is known as the fetal ejection reflex. It helps babies to birth quickly and easily and stimulates the initiation of infant respiration. The combination of adrenaline and oxytocin at birth creates the wide-eyed, alert, and focused gaze we associate with newborns. After birth, levels of adrenaline quickly drop. For birthing women this can result in a cold, shaky feeling for a short while after birth.

When the neocortex is resting and the primal brain takes charge, endorphins and oxytocin are released into the system. Endorphins are the "feel-good" hormones we produce for pain relief, which are morphine like in their makeup and intensity. Endorphins are secreted by the pituitary gland, and high levels are present during pregnancy, labor, and birth. Endorphins are potent painkillers, and if the endorphin level is very high during labor it can somewhat inhibit the production of oxytocin. This would, therefore, reduce the intensity of the pain experienced for a while.

Endorphins also help our babies to adapt to extra-uterine life. According to Charles D. Laughlin, "The sudden release of endorphins prior to birth may have a regulatory effect upon respiration after birth (Moss 1986), and may well be a factor in producing the experience had by the fetus/neonate during a 'natural' birth."[26] Birth adrenaline is quickly passed through the babies' systems, and the pleasure-inducing endorphins that have entered their systems from placental transfer during labor help to settle our babies into their new and very strange world. Endorphins are also present in breast milk.

Oxytocin stimulates and controls the great uterine surges that open the cervix, and it also promotes bonding by causing a feeling of intense love. Oxytocin is produced at birth and during orgasm, and, depending on the circumstances, the love is either directed at our partners or at our babies.

Hormones influence our emotions. These hormones attach to receptor sites in the cells of our bodies, causing us to perceive events from a particular emotional outlook. Birth—as every mother knows—is a time of mega hormone production. The hypothalamus is set on overdrive, and our emotions are often topsy-turvy. Once our controling, analytical brain gets out the way, our primal, intuitive brain can guide the birth process. So, the more animal-like we become, the easier the labor and birth usually are. Laboring in the dreamlike state brought on by deep immersion into the limbic brain is the most powerful way to produce oxytocin and endorphins. Undisturbed births usually help bonding occur naturally and instinctively. Hormone production influences not only the labor but also the bonding process after birth. In the postpartum period we continue to produce oxytocin, which keeps us relaxed and de-stressed. It is also the hormone associated with love and helps with bonding.

Hospital birth practices that intervene in the natural process of birth, such as induction, augmentation, epidurals, pain-relieving drugs, Caesarean section, immediate cutting of the umbilical cord after birth, and separation of us from our babies after birth, all have the potential to upset our ability to produce hormones that aid us in our birthing. These hormones give us a sense of extraordinary achievement post birth and create optimum conditions for bonding and breast-feeding.

Fetal experience

" In short, intra-uterine bonding does not happen automatically: Love for the child and understanding of one's own feelings are needed to make it work. When these are present, they can more than offset the emotional disturbances we are all prone to in our daily lives. "

—*Dr. Thomas Verny, Expert on prenatal personality development* [27]

Until recently it was believed that babies only began to feel, think, and dream after birth. However, recent evidence shows that not only is the birth often traumatic and crucial in forming life patterns but that prenatal experience is also formative to future life. [28]

As a result of studies undertaken by prenatal and perinatal psychologists, scientists are now conceding that babies in utero respond to complex biochemical influences (and, therefore, to their mother's emotional state), and to environmental influences such as movement, light, and sound. An international congress of prenatal and perinatal psychology of North America was established in the 1980s, and researchers such as Dr. Stanislav Grof and many others have made important contributions to this field of inquiry.

The fetus has been found to be immensely sensitive and capable. This discovery has become very apparent with the advent of ultrasound scanning, where the baby's movements can be clearly observed. Amniocentesis, for example, is performed at the same time as ultrasound these days, and the fetus can often be seen to withdraw from the intrusion of the needle into the amniotic fluid. Benig Mauger describes a fetus that was seen to attack the needle with his fist a few times.[29] Parents often describe an ultrasound of their unborn as a delightful event, not least because their baby was sucking its thumb or scratching its head. These activities are obviously chosen and are not simply reflex actions.

Not only do babies in the womb partake of activities for pleasure, they also react to unpleasant situations, even to emotionally unpleasant situations. In a study undertaken in the United States, Correia measured the effect on the fetus of a mother viewing brief portions of a violent movie. The fetus was as upset as the mother.[30] It makes rational sense that this should be so, since we know that the mother's hormones, that is endorphins or adrenaline, pass through the placental barrier.

Babies are also sensitive to our emotions. This statement has the potential to engender feelings of guilt. Almost every one of us has moments during pregnancy when we are irritated, angry, feel ugly, unhappy, or stressed out from work. Unplanned babies often experience an adjustment period when their parents are adapting to the idea of having them, and when they may even be clearly unwanted for a while.

According to Dr. Thomas Verny in *The Secret Life of the Unborn Child*, continued stress, particularly when linked to our partners, can be damaging to the emotional security of a child. However, short periods of stress are not likely to be problematic,[31] and most of us experience at least some of that in our pregnancies, particularly in first pregnancies, when all sorts of unexpected adaptations to our situation arise and when it slowly begins to dawn on us what having a baby really means in terms of lifestyle changes. If our emotions have long-term impacts on our unborn children, it seems virtually impossible for us not to harm them. This is earth, after all. I believe I chose to come here. Sometimes when I'm feeling down, I entertain myself with the idea that perhaps I could have chosen heaven instead. But here I am, and my parents, my children, and I all have to get along with that and deal with the imperfections I carry in my earthly form.

We know that the senses of unborn babies develop early on in the pregnancy. As early as six or seven weeks in utero, the baby has body chemicals in place that carry messages throughout its system.[32] By the time it is fully developed, the fetus has all its senses, except perhaps smell, operating within its womb environment. They develop in the following order:

Touch: The first sense to be developed is the sense of touch. Reflexes to direct sensory stimulation begin between seven and eight weeks of gestation. The baby will respond to unpleasant sensations. Between the eleventh and twelfth weeks it moves its face away from a stimulus. At fourteen weeks it can be seen to frown and grimace. By seventeen weeks, it shows a definite sensitivity to touch in all parts of its body.

Taste: The unborn baby sips amniotic fluid from twelve weeks on. Amniotic fluid contains protein and sugar. At two months, taste buds appear in the fetal mouth. When a bitter substance is injected into the amniotic fluid, investigators have observed a baby stop drinking or swallowing. Babies also drink more when saccharine is introduced.[33]

Sight: From the sixteenth week onward, the unborn child is sensitive to light. The light inside the uterus is perceived as a warm red glow. Bright light shone onto the womb causes a startled reaction; gentle light causes the baby to turn toward it slowly.[34] Between thirty-two and thirty-six weeks, there are strong responses to light and sound.

Hearing: The baby is highly sound-sensitized by twenty-five weeks. Amniotic fluid is a more effective sound conductor than air, so the child hears the mother's pulse, her digestive noises, and her heartbeat. Newborns are comforted by tape recordings of their mother's heartbeat. Babies have been observed to react positively to Brahms and Vivaldi, while reacting with violent kicking motions to loud rock music. Newborns recognize not only their mother's voice but also that of their father's, especially if the father has been talking to the child in the womb.[35] Unborn babies tend to be gentled by low-frequency sounds and agitated by high-frequency ones. A Doppler, the fetal heart monitor that midwives use to listen to the baby's heartbeat, increases fetal heart rate, while an ultrasound does not.[36]

Interestingly, in a study by medical researcher Peter Hepper, newborn babies have been noted to recognize theme tunes from soap operas, which their mothers watched frequently while carrying them. Perhaps because they are a reminder of their womb days, these theme tunes seem to have a remarkably calming effect on babies whose mothers watched the soap operas, while having no visible effect on a control group of babies who were not exposed to prenatal television.[37]

Rosario N. Rozada reported in "Singing Lullabies to Unborn Children: Experiences in Village Vilamarxant"[38] that "[when] pregnant women began singing, clapping, tapping with their hands and feet in performing folk songs and lullabies for two hours a week, they discovered a cascade of psychological benefits, including emotional expression, tension relief, and a powerful group solidarity. Their babies seemed to join them, too. Two older mothers scheduled for Caesareans gave birth spontaneously and confidently. After the babies were born, mothers found themselves more proficient at calming their neonates to sleep and were able to breast-feed longer."

It is now apparent that a child's emotional development also begins in the womb. Not only sound vibrations but a mother's fatigue level and emotions also affect her unborn child. It is not the occasional and normal tension and worry of everyday life that causes serious problems, but

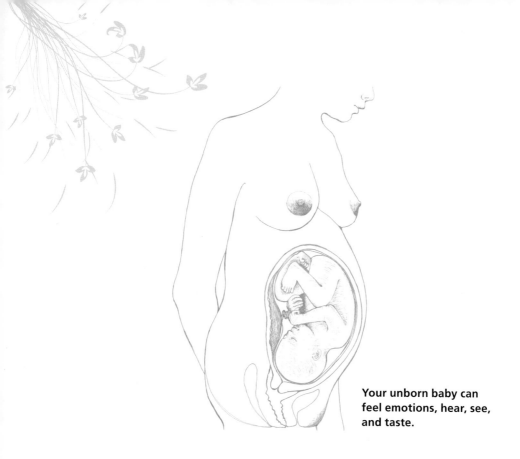

Your unborn baby can feel emotions, hear, see, and taste.

rather chronic and continuous stress experienced by the mother that has been found to cause problems. Stress hormones are secreted under chronic stress conditions, which may adversely affect the fetus.[39]

In another very interesting study conducted by Dr. Michael Lieberman, it was discovered that a baby's heartbeat would increase before its mother lit a cigarette, in anticipation of the actual smoking.[40] Explanations for this include the possibility of the mother's own heartbeat increasing in anticipation of the cigarette, or that adrenaline crosses the placental barrier and stimulates the fetal heart.

Freud suggested that the prenatal state was characterized "by an oceanic feeling of bliss." However, pre- and perinatal psychology are now discovering that this may not always be so. Regression therapy indicates that the womb is also a place where it is possible to suffer.

My personal experience of assisting people to regress back into womb states, bears both Freud's and the regressionist theories. While the experiences of numerous people may have been difficult or traumatic (an example of a traumatic prenatal experience could be the recognition that the mother does not want this pregnancy), the perspective from which these experiences are viewed is very objective. There is invariably a deep understanding of the purpose of the experience, as well as empathy for their parents. Adults who re-experience life in the womb (and are viewing it from the fetal perspective) have an ability to see beyond their pain, to understand the purpose of it. The prenatal child, it seems, is still cushioned in an ego-free state. Confirmation of this might be demonstrated when considering how babies move gradually from the stage where they are not ego-dominated to the stage of being self-conscious, demanding two-year-olds. Premature babies seem to have an energy that is wise beyond our adult understanding of wisdom, an archetypal, collective wisdom, that does not belong to them personally.

People undergoing regression also view miscarriages, abortions, and threatened mis-carriages as decisions, that are made on a super-conscious level by both the child and the parents. There never seem to be "mistakes." Leni Schwartz writes, in *Bonding before Birth*, that it is now understood that child and mother influence each other, both biologically and emotionally.

In *Expecting Adam*, an autobiography of a mother who bore a Down's syndrome child, Martha Beck describes the experiences of her pregnancy and birth, and of how telepathi-cally linked she was to her unborn child. The baby communicated with her through dreams, visions, and intuitive thought. This was remarkable to her because she considered herself to be a prime example of a rational, logical individual, with three degrees from Harvard University. She began her pregnancy as someone who required that facts should be empiri-cally tested and provable to be able to fit into her worldview; yet she was forced to radically expand her concept of reality, thanks to the prodding of her baby.[41] We set out to prove that babies can learn in the womb, only to discover that perhaps they know more than us, and perhaps we are the ones capable of learning from the experience.

The research that has been done to prove that the fetus is a conscious being has pro-found psychological, emotional, and social significance for our treatment of our babies within our wombs. If we are honored and respected as wise and conscious beings within the womb, then it could have an enormous impact on our behavior in society, postnatally, and on our sense of self-esteem.

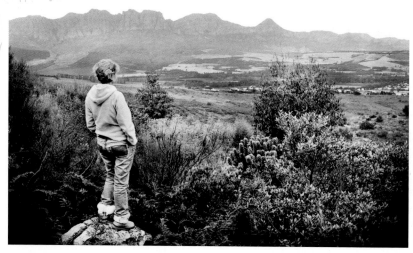

Karen

Karen's birth story

 The beginning is present in the end.

—Sufi saying

My child's birth, against expectations, was in almost every aspect an exact replica of the abortion I had had thirteen years before that. I was talked into the abortion by my boyfriend. I was so young, twenty, and being pregnant was such a shocking thing in my family. They were very conservative. In some ways the abortion was the easy way out, so I allowed my boyfriend to overrule me, even though I knew in my heart of hearts that I wanted to keep the child. I was just so scared of facing my parents with the news. So my boyfriend flew me to Durban where there was a woman trained by a gynecologist to do it properly. When she injected me with this stuff one half of me became paralysed and the other half was in labor. So it ended up being a very traumatic experience. Because abortions were illegal, the woman wanted to give herself up at the police station so that I could be taken to hospital. It was traumatic. When the little thing finally came down it was still in the sac, warm against my legs. I was haunted for years by the memory of the warmth of that little body.

Afterwards, all hell broke loose inside me. My heart was broken. I had no idea that the whole experience would turn out to be so traumatic. I started blaming myself that I had killed someone, my own child. Deep depressions took me. I started dreaming about this child. In my dreams, I would have conversations with him and play with him at night. It was my consolation for years. It was also my spiritual awakening, because the realization that maybe I had committed an unforgivable thing broke me open into searching for what was the truth behind all the rules of society, behind all the concepts of good and bad. I was willing to let go of my belief systems, anything, for the sake of finding the truth. There was a huge longing released inside me, and I can only describe it as the longing to see what is beyond this reality, and find the Divine reality. I realized much later that in a way Jack came to wake me up. This was the gift he brought to me in this life.

After the abortion it was impossible to live with who I was. I explored any possible way to work through my traumas and to find ways into the Real, that which is hidden behind every concept and structure of this world. Every year around the 15th of June—the day of the abortion—I wanted to kill myself. Sometimes I felt it, without realizing it was that date again. Nine years after the abortion, on the 15th of June, I went into a cathedral. All I wanted was to sit in silence and burn a candle. In one corner stood a big Madonna carved from black wood, in intimate union with her baby. His skin glowed like a polished brown nut.

Then I heard the voice of the child I knew so well from my dreams. It spoke from inside me. "Can you see how the Madonna and her child are carved from the same block of wood? They are one. We are the same. You never lost me. We are woven together, you and I. Now stop tormenting yourself. All is forgiven."

In the years up until then, I had done penance and here he was setting me free. For years ten, eleven, and twelve, on the 15th of June, I didn't have the suicide blues anymore.

When I heard about the due date for Jack's birth, I never thought about the fact that it was a week before the date that the abortion occurred thirteen years before. I was surprised afterward that I did not think of the date, really. I had no expectations that he would be born on that day, probably because the inner work was done. But when he came, it was in a way that was so clear it was the same child, the same date, the same physical conditions. It just stormed through my senses.

I didn't dilate properly. I'd wanted a water birth but had to be taken to hospital. >

The contractions were not regular and went on for hours. Something in me became so totally in tune that when the anesthetist finally walked in, I looked up and said "You're not going to only do one half of my body are you?" But that is exactly what happened. Just like thirteen years before in the abortion, half of my body was paralyzed and the other half had to give birth and the whole thing became traumatic and painful. Jack was lying with his spine against my spine—an occiput posterior position, which is more painful.

Once again his water didn't break; it only happened as he was born. When he finally slipped out I felt that longed-for warmth of the life in him against my thighs, and something in me snapped out of the expecting-death mode that I was in. Of course, nothing could have prepared me for that moment when I first saw him. None of the above reasons why I know it was the same soul, measured up to that moment of recognition. When I looked at him, when our eyes locked in at that moment, it carried such power. I couldn't believe it. He came out—deep, deep blue eyes looking into my eyes—and there was this moment of 'Oh my sweet Lord, it's you!' Until that moment in my life, I had never experienced such love. It was such a shock to love like that. It was inconceivable until that moment that it could be like that. For this being I was willing to give everything, to walk over hot coals, to be sliced in pieces, whatever it took.

I felt my arms reach out to him, as if they were empty and longing for hundreds of years. It was like a long, slow-motion moment in which I reached over an ancient longing and unfulfillment, and then he was in my arms. We had made it through together this time. I just snapped into bliss and a joy that I will never be able to capture in words. Here was the little warm creature I had wanted to hold for so long, safely back in my arms. And he had turned the destiny of my soul.

If he had slipped out in the water at home, and the birth had been all perfectly easy and spiritual and la-di-dah, I could have had some doubts whether it was the same child. But for some reason destiny took over, and he was born with almost everything "going wrong" in the same way as the abortion.

And it happened on the same day, the 15th of June, thirteen years later.

The birth happening in this unplanned way was also about my dreams being shattered. It broke my illusions of how birth should happen and how motherhood should be. And again as a baby, as a child, he always challenged my beliefs of what was good and right and spiritual, so eventually I would become surrendered to what life needed, not what I thought was better.

Looking back at it, I can see how perfectly it was designed. Nothing else could have driven me through the difficulties of the years ahead. But this love could. It was a love I did not feel for myself. It took this child to catapult me into the depths of the transformation that was to come.

On a soul level there was the indescribable experience of forgiveness that came along with this birth. It felt as if divine forces smiled on me and gave me back what I had thrown away in a heedless moment, when I was young. The abortion was an act that would haunt me for so many years, but it was the lead in the alchemist's crucible of love that would have to eventually become transformed.

After his birth, I had the same experience of it being impossible to live with who I was. Because he was pure essence, he showed up all my childhood trauma. That love—how do I put this?—was so enormous that when I realized the pain that the child was in afterward because of his colic and the hunger when my breast milk dried up from the stress, the love and the understanding that he and I are reflections, are parts of each other, and that I'm responsible for his suffering, drove me to transform myself for his sake, and my whole life has been about transformation. I would not have transformed for my own sake. But it was the single most horrifying thing to see this little being suffer and know that I was responsible.

Slowly I came to realize through the years that what was in my shadow, in my unconscious, would be played out by my child unless I transformed first. When Jack hit the age where I was when my childhood abuse happened, he activated my inner child's pain. And it was like waving a magic wand. If he was sick, I would work on myself, face my own pain, face what I didn't want to face in my own psyche, and he would heal. Over and over and over this would happen.

In my essence being exposed to his essence, all my childhood memories of abuse came up, because they weren't essence; they were part of the wound. And I realized the only way to communicate with Jack was in a completely different way, which had nothing to do with how I was parented. If I didn't communicate from essence to essence, from my heart to his heart, in vulnerability and honesty yet standing my ground, I lost his trust, I lost the gentle flow and magic between us, and it would fall into the old patterns of parenting, where the child is forced to resist and live out the parent's shadow.

The Sufis have a term called the 'Tauber,' which means a turning of the heart, that usually an 'enlightened' week or two that changes your direction in life. After seeing >

that truth, having had a glimpse of what is real, you have the driving force to trans-mute all the human illusion. And I always wondered, what was my Tauber? For me it was not an experience of bliss; it was first the abortion and the deep seeking of truth it opened up in me, and then this birth of my child and my love for him. Both these events turned the key. There was nothing ever in my life that would make me want to have had these experiences differently. It was one of the most profound things, along with being abused by my dad, which drove me to start living the true purpose of my life. It ignited the longing for God, to live another reality, and I had so many belief sys-tems to let go of.

It forced me to face my shadow, face myself, and take full responsibility for my life. This is one of the most difficult things for a human being to do, and I would not have done it if I did not feel so tortured. I am so deeply grateful for my son and my father, the one through being his pure self, and the other through being his tortured self, for having given me the courage, the incentive, to do what needed to be done.

BIRTH
CHOICES

Chapter Three

> "You are constructing your own reality with the choices you make...
> or don't make. If you really want a healthy pregnancy and joyful
> birth, and you truly understand that you are the one in control, then
> you must examine what you have or haven't done so far to create
> the outcome you want. "
>
> — *Kim Wildner, Hypnotherapist* [42]

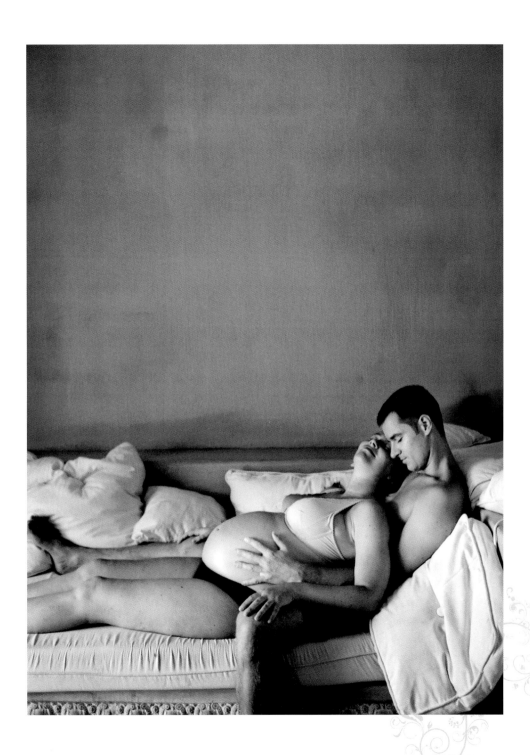

Birth choices

" Given the opportunity to voice their opinions about what
is happening in their labor and how their baby is doing,
women will often give you a very accurate account.
The key is to listen to them. "

— *Jill Cohen, Associate editor Midwifery Today Magazine* [43]

Birth belongs to the woman who is laboring and to her baby who is being born, not to the caregivers who are monitoring them. Emotional and spiritual preparation during pregnancy creates a clear birthing vision for mother and baby. This increases the likelihood that both mother and baby will be awake, alert, and hormonally primed for bonding in those precious first hours following the birth.

Laboring women perceive their birth as satisfying or not, largely according to whether they are consulted in the decisions made around how their labor should progress. The more informed women are prior to their labor, the easier it is for them to make choices that they feel are in the best interests of their babies. Women who are involved in the decision-making process during their labors and birthings are generally the women who are most content with their birth outcomes.

Birth from a baby's perspective

" And the end of all our exploring will be to arrive where we started
and know the place for the first time. "

— *T. S. Eliot, Poet and Nobel Prize winner*

Birth serves as a bridge between being a woman and becoming a mother. In many ways this massive shift on all levels of our being is supported by the intensity of the birth experience. Women who disconnect from the experience through Caesarean births, epidurals (akin to watching telly during labor), or through fear of the process of normal birth, could potentially rob themselves of one of the most meaningful life events. If we are to honor the baby's part in the process of labor and birth, this would include allowing him to choose the time of his birth, and letting go of the need to control the environment around us during birth so that we can be more fully present in each moment.

If babies could talk and write at birth, a few would probably be out there, protesting for their downtrodden contemporaries, no doubt with slogans like "Get undressed, we want more breast" or "Mom and Dad and Sis, a family bed is bliss." Babies are so non-judgmental and accepting of circumstances, though, that they've left it up to us to protest on their behalf. It seems that babies don't hold onto conscious memory of traumatic events; instead these memories are stored in the unconscious mind, where their impact creates a subtle change in perception of the world they live in.

The reason we don't remember our births is that we have not yet developed selfconscious awareness. Memory is stored in the section of our brains that is selfconscious, which usually only begins developing at around two years of age. Our awareness at birth is interdependent with the awareness of the "other." If my perception is that I am my mother, her moods and certainly her disconnection from me affect my perception of the world and cause me emotional and perhaps even physical pain.

Before birth, research shows that babies are already aware within the watery world of their wombs. If unborn babies are so aware of their environment, traditional cultures can remind us to be more conscious of the emotional impact that pregnancy, labor, and birth have on them. Often cultural taboos surrounding birth stem from a baby's need for gentle adjustment into the world. Batswana women, for example, historically spent the first three months postpartum cloistered in the birth room, bonding with their baby, eating soft porridge, tended by only one or two women caregivers.

Many obstetricians and midwives these days have never seen a baby who is not mildly shocked at birth. Not knowing what they're not seeing they expect babies to have a stunned and distressed expression at birth; therefore they are not questioning if there is another way. However, babies born naturally, without interference, with full attention, patience, and an undisturbed, warm welcome are likely to be alert, curious, and trusting.

Provided everybody is healthy, the atmosphere created by the parents and participants at the birth is as important as the physical environment. A satisfying birth to one mother may be an epidural or elective Caesarean, while to another it may be giving birth in the woods, under the stars, with no one but one's husband and kids in attendance. Satisfied mothers often produce satisfied babies.

Take my friend Jen's babies, for example. They're both gorgeous. She gave birth both times in hospital, the first with an ineffective epidural, the second with an overwhelmingly intense, albeit short, induced birth. They were born into bright lights, hospital noise, and a clinically sterile environment. However, they were longed for, adored, and doted

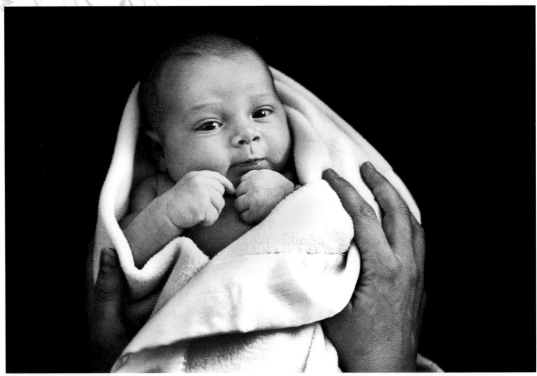

Birth is a baby's first experience of life. It impacts strongly on how deeply they trust the world. Their primary need is to feel your attention and welcome at this moment.

upon. I visited Jen the morning after the birth of Dale, her firstborn. She looked pale, exhausted, and shaky. I asked how she was feeling and while still unable to tear her eyes away from him, she answered that she was very tired, but hadn't been able to close her eyes yet, since they had been gazing at each other all night. Both of Jen's kids are self-assured, and for now at least, sit happily, chubbily, and solidly in their small bodies.

Helping newborns settle into their bodies requires an awareness of all these different layers of experience going on for them, much of which we've become desensitized to. On a physical level they need to adjust to breathing through their lungs, which is scary when they don't know how yet, and their oxygen supply from the umbilical cord has been severed. On a more sensitive level, sounds, smells, and sights are strident after the muffled atmosphere inside the belly. Babies like familiarity to help them adjust to their new environment.

Recreating womb like surroundings helps to soothe newborns. A mother who feels a close connection to her baby at birth will often naturally want to create a place with soft sounds and dim lights that is private and personal enough for getting to know each other. Reimmersing babies in water soon after birth, placing them close to their mother's heartbeat, feeling their body close to hers, keeping them at a temperature close to that of amniotic fluid, and swaddling them as a reminder of the contained space of the womb, all help to overcome the shock of such a huge new world. Then deep down and supporting the other layers, is the subtler, more unconscious level of "vibes" surrounding the birth. Parents are often finely tuned in to these feelings in the weeks after birth, but babies can't avoid them since they don't yet have the emotional barriers set up to keep an unpleasant atmosphere at bay.

I have seen a seven-week-old premature baby smiling in an incubator, and incubators are unfriendly, lonely places when your primary needs are for love, nourishment, and security. However, she was adored by her mother, and something about her situation felt more healing than an epidural birth I attended, where the parents, though delighted by the pain-freelabor, were watching cricket on the telly within half an hour of this seeming non-event. Did they want me to switch the TV off? Absolutely not, it was a test match!

Birth choices are individual and should be made to suit varying needs. However, if the choices are to be infant—rather than mother—based, the bottom line, perhaps, is that a baby's most primal need at birth is for undiluted, undisturbed love. Babies then require warmth, security, and nourishment. Occasionally, a newly birthed baby needs medical attention to get started. As with us adults, though, in the birth room it seems that it is the simple pleasures that matter most. Ultimately, it is love that helps a newborn find their way home.

Over-medicated birth

" According to the medical model, life is a problem because it is full of risk and in almost constant danger, an assumption easily accepted if one's professional career is spent surrounded by pathology, suffering, and death. "

— Marsden Wagner, MD - Pediatrician and perinatologist [44]

I am very grateful to Lisa who gave birth to Jade yesterday afternoon. She slipped into this book just ten days prior to it going to print. Lisa had birthed her previous child, Michael, by Caesarean section after a long labor. This had had a negative emotional impact on her. She felt robbed of the experience of natural birth and was concerned that Michael hadn't had the best initial experience of life. So she desperately wanted Jade to have a natural birth, and she put an immense amount of work into her birth preparation.

She trained in deep relaxation techniques, she attended movement and mindfulness classes for pregnancy, she practiced prenatal yoga, relaxation, and exercise. She ate well and healthily. She explored process work, using art and dance to look at her fears. She and her husband both attended dance class for working with creating an intimate atmosphere for birth, and both took part in a session of connecting with Jade as an unborn child to receive her guidance for how she would like her birth to be.

Incidentally, during this session, they asked Michael to take a symbolic form and to describe the effect that his birth had had on him. He took the form of a whale, with huge energy, that simply couldn't be squashed through the birth canal. Lisa visualized him needing to leap out of her womb by Caesarean birth, and during the session he expressed that his birth was exactly the way he had intended it to be.

By the time she was ready to give birth; Lisa was looking forward to the event and mentioned that she felt quite saturated with birth preparations. She had asked me to be her labor attendant to help her with employing her birth preparation techniques during labor. Sue was her midwife. She had a planned hospital birth because she was intending to have a VBAC—Vaginal Birth After Caesarean—and her obstetrician wanted her to be close to the operating theater.

After ten hours of active labor Lisa was fully dilated; yet, Jade never came close to descending into her pelvis prior to moving down through the birth canal. During the labor, Jade had turned from an occiput anterior to an occiput posterior position, which means she was face forwards—a more difficult position to birth in. An occiput posterior position in labor can be an indication that the pelvis is a tight fit, and Jade may have been trying different positions because the normal and easiest one wasn't working well. As a VBAC, there was a limited amount of time that Lisa was given for the pushing stage. Too long and too intense a second stage after a previous Caesarean birth can lead to prob-lems or at worst, possible rupture of the uterine scar. So Lisa tried with all her might to push Jade out into the world and that was that with natural birth for her. We all agreed that Jade was going to have to find an alternative route into the world, and like Michael, she was finally born by Caesarean section.

I realized I had been invested in her having a natural birth because she had wanted it so badly and had worked so hard for it; yet, Jade's birth didn't work out that way. For Lisa, it didn't in any way feel like a failure. Half an hour after birth Jade was very calm. She loved breastfeeding, and she was snuggling up to Lisa. Lisa looked tired and relaxed, like someone who had achieved a wonderful birth, because she had done everything that she could to make it so. Jade's birth choices, while not those Lisa would have chosen, had been ones she fully agreed were in their best interests. It even felt wonderful that they had experienced the long and arduous labor instead of an elective Caesarean birth. She says, *"Labor was a heal-ing experience for me, and a powerful deepening of Cliff's and my relationship. I felt that he really went into the fire with me. I feel deep peace knowing that I did my best. That we all did. And it has reconciled me with the course that Michael's birth took, too. In the end, we are blessed with two healthy, beautiful children, and I am filled with gratitude that all our caregivers showed such profound commitment to support my wish to deliver Jade naturally, and in the end to ensure both of our safety and health. Jade's birth confirmed for me that birth and parenthood are a lot about surrender, and as Sue wisely reminded me at my post-natal visit, 'Its not always just about you.'"*

Lisa sits here in this book as a testament that birth is the way it is. She is an admirable example of the truth that the best births for our children are not necessarily those that we would choose for them. I love that Lisa is here, in this book, a quiet and courageous reminder that we simply do what we can and that birth, like life, is not perfect.

Nevertheless, we seem to be free-falling into a 21st-century mode of producing our babies using medical interventions as our primary birth option. Caesarean birth rates are ris-ing annually, and induction rates have never been higher. Our power to give birth according to our body's wisdom is eroding at an exponential rate.

We watch television channels dedicated to depicting horrifying birth stories. We exchange tales of episiotomy pain. The nightmares of labor, of our reliance on the medical profession to save us from the nightmare. And we forget, each time a little more, that this is not the way it was meant to be.

Many children born these days are second-generation babies who have been surgically removed from their mothers at birth, pulled out into cold, harsh lights in operating theaters, with little welcome, in fact little *notice* paid to their intensely sensitive, emotional, and spiritual well-being. Bonding is often delayed, breastfeeding disparaged, welcoming rituals all but forgotten. If we ever question the emotional state of our world, and wonder about the harshness of it, we naturally arrive at birth as the first insult on our emotional well-being. Birth may very well have been the first time we had to close down our emotional field in order to cope with intense stress.

Many obstetricians are failing to alert and inform women fully of the potential outcomes of intervening in a normal, uncomplicated birth. [See information on Caesareans on pages 87–98, and their references on page 261 in the endnotes.] Women are sometimes persuaded, for non-medical reasons, to opt for a Caesarean or an induction. The "your baby is too big" reason too often produces babies who are average, sometimes even below average, in weight.

These babies survive and carry on to lead normal lives in our rushed and stressed-out world. But who is querying the long-term national and global impact that births with so little warmth and gentleness and patience are having on our societies, our cultures, our human experience?

A woman experiencing a natural birth in a supportive environment produces hormones that properly encourage the baby to adapt to life outside the womb in a less traumatized fashion. Babies who enter the world in an unhurried way, slipping out into their mother's embrace where they are quietly taken care of and loved, are more relaxed in their bodies and may be calmer and less fretful in their first few months. Birth makes an impact on the newborn psyche in either a positive or negative way. Each time a woman makes clearly informed decisions in the best interests of her baby's physical, emotional, and spiritual well-being, she is empowering those who follow her to do the same.

Nevertheless, Caesarean births play a very important role in birth in the 21st-century. In about 7 per-cent of births, Caesarians are hugely beneficial. They save lives and keep us and our babies safe, and they provide a secure environment so that we can trust that labor is not a life-threatening process. Women may choose to birth by Caesarean section; what is important is that their birth choices are not taken away from them unnecessarily.

Place of birth

Where you choose to birth is important in terms of the type of experience you are likely to have. Consider what the options are in the area in which you live, and visit or interview the caregivers who work in each.

Home birth

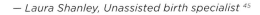

Privacy is as essential to birth as it is to sex.

— *Laura Shanley, Unassisted birth specialist* [45]

Home birth may be perceived as satisfying. There are several reasons for this. Home-birth midwives are generally dedicated, supportive, and caring, having already built up a trusting relationship with the parents; the atmosphere at a home birth is usually relaxed and peaceful; and the courage required by the mother to stand up for such choices in the face of an often-critical society and medical community means that she makes her birth choices with great care.

There have been many studies comparing the safety of home birth with low-risk hospital birth. The most recent research, published in the BMJ (British Medical Journal), was a North American study of 5,418 women who opted for home births supported by CPMs (Certified Professional Midwives). The study compared their perinatal outcomes with birth statistics from the birth certificates of comparable low-risk hospital births in the United States during the same time period.[46]

Notable results of the study include:

- Rates of medical interventions (including electronic fetal monitoring, episiotomy, Caesarean birth, and vacuum extraction) were consistently less than half of those found in hospital samples.
- No maternal deaths occurred in the intrapartum period.
- The neonatal mortality rate was 1.7 deaths per 1,000 low-risk planned home births, which is consistent with other studies of planned birth center births and low-risk hospital births in North America.

A certified professional midwife will usually take the equivalent of a labor ward to a home birth. Oxygen, a suction machine, drugs for managing complications of birth, and fetal monitoring equipment are fairly standard labor accessories at a home birth. Often the midwife will call an assistant to help her in the final stages of the birth, so that two pairs of hands are available to look after both mother and baby should that be necessary. To keep birth safety optimal, it is important to organize a backup obstetrician who agrees to be on call should you require an emergency Caesarean birth.

Home birth is one of those jobs that midwives decide to do because they love birth and because they believe that their clients have the best chance of surrendering into birth at home. In countries that have a strong focus on the medicalization of birth, such as the United States and South Africa, midwives have to be strong enough to withstand pressure from the medical community to conform to their beliefs about controling birth. This atmosphere creates responsible groups of independent midwives who truly believe in a woman's right to choose how she would like to give birth.

I have often heard obstetricians and hospital-based midwives question why women would take the chance of birthing away from the security of theaters, obstetricians, and pediatricians, simply to have their babies at home. They can't see the point. I attend births both at home and in hospitals, and I understand that the point of home birth could be missed if you've never attended one. The difference is subtle, but it is also very deep. It arises from our attitudes, intentions, and approach to birth. At home, it's easier to be aware of how important love and support is in the birthing equation for mothers, fathers, and their babies. I notice the difference in the babies, who are less likely to find birth shocking and who are often very quiet, peaceful, and alert. Parents too, are often transformed by the experience of home birth.

Birth centers

Birth centers may suit women who choose an atmosphere that is more like a home birth, with the security of hospital technology close by. Water births are often available, along with water immersion after birth for the baby. At a birth center serving the Hispanic community on the American side of the US-Mexico border, where I worked for a while, the babies were often immersed in warm water shortly after birth. They would visibly unwind and relax, and obviously found the familiar feeling soothing and calming.

Birth centers are created to offer women the midwifery model of care as opposed to the medical model of care. This midwifery model of care is described by *Childbirth Connection* (www.childbirthconnection.org) in the following manner:

Midwifery Model of Care
- Care focuses on health, wellness, prevention
- Labor/birth are seen as normal physiological processes
- Lower rates of using interventions
- Mother gives birth
- Care is individualized

Medical Model of Care
- Care focuses on managing problems and complications
- Labor/birth are dependent on technology
- Higher rates of using interventions
- Doctor delivers baby
- Care is routinized

"Naturally, the midwifery model describes the practice of many midwives, and the medical model describes the practice of many doctors. But many caregivers combine elements of both. It is possible, but less common, to find doctors whose practice most closely resembles the midwifery model of care and midwives whose practice most closely resembles the medical model. The Midwives Model of Care is based on the premise that pregnancy and birth are normal life processes."[47]

Hospital births

Most women in the First World give birth in hospital, very often with an obstetrician in attendance. It is our responsibility as women to ensure that we know the consequences of refusing pain relief, pethidine, epidurals, inductions, or Caesarean births.

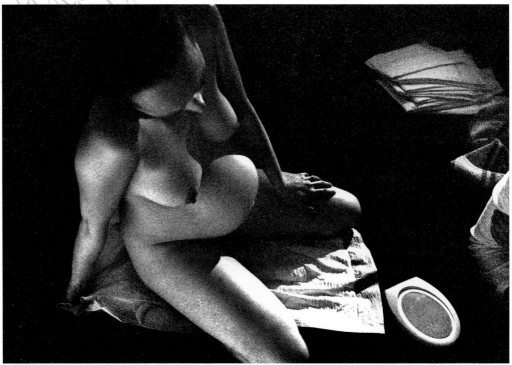

We have millions of years of intuitive knowing held in our DNA and the cells of our bodies about how to give birth vaginally We need only learn to trust this knowing.

Types of birth

Vaginal birth

> " The way to prevent episiotomies is not to do them. "
>
> — *Katherine Jensen* [48]

Many women assume that they will be giving birth vaginally, only to find that they are persuaded differently for a variety of factors, many of which are not necessarily in their or their babies' best interests. If you plan a vaginal birth, depending on where you live, it may be necessary for you to discuss this in some detail with your prospective caregiver during the first half of your pregnancy, so that you can make birth choices that support your wishes. (See interview guidelines on page 99.)

Caesarean birth

A Caesarean section can be traumatic for a baby, but this is dramatically reduced if his parents give him immediate love and attention, and if the early bonding period is disturbed as little as possible. Sometimes a woman will require a Caesarean as a medical necessity, and this is a time to be grateful for their availability. According to the World Health Organization, the most beneficial outcomes for mother and baby happen when the Caesarean birth rate in a country is between 7–10%. Less than this has dire consequences in terms of morbidity and mortality, especially in Third World countries with poor living conditions and only the most basic medical facilities. When the rate drops below 2 percent, the outcomes plummet. However, in South Africa, in the private sector, we have a Caesarean birth rate of more than 70 percent.

Many obstetricians would have us believe that Caesarean births are safer for mothers and babies. The statistics simply do not bear this out. Rather than attributing improved birth statistics and mortality rates over the past decades to the increase in Caesarean birth rates, they should be attributed to the privilege of available Caesareans when they are medically warranted, the availability of Neonatal Intensive Care Units, improved nutrition and prenatal care, and the availability of abortions.

When I was asked to talk on the subject at a midwifery conference last year, I was given the opportunity to research what the high rate of Caesarean births in South African private hospitals meant in terms of birth outcomes. The sometimes shocking research results quoted below are comparing women who give birth in First World countries. They do not include statistics from countries that have little or no medical support for birthing women, poor nutritional standards, and high rates of socio economic distress. All the studies quoted here have been systematically reviewed and rated on a scale of one to five; one being randomized controled trials, five being narrative studies. Only levels one to three were included in the data.

Most of the studies were drawn from research undertaken by a team led by Dr Carol Sakala, who analyzed more than three hundred studies comparing Caesarean birth and vaginal birth outcomes, the only one of its kind to date. The review was used to produce an educational booklet, which has been endorsed by thirty organisations promoting maternal infant health: *What Every Pregnant Woman Needs to Know About Cesarean Section.*[49] A worrying statistic that has been found in the United States during the past decade is the ongoing increase in low birth-weight babies and in preterm births. There are concerns that this may be due to the escalating number of elective deliveries in healthy women.

References for the studies that the following statistics were drawn from are available in the endnotes at the back of the book. If you choose to pass any of this information onto your caregiver, it will be necessary to include the references.

Caregivers rely on evidence-based research in providing guidelines for quality care; however, we need to be scrupulous in our analysis of the studies and to recognize their limitations. Trials are expensive to run and need sponsorship, often from large corporations. As a result, fewer studies are undertaken that seek to prove that natural birth is a healthy option than those that prove the efficacy of drugs or intervention techniques using modern equipment. The quality and size of the study should be checked, as should the parameters within which it is based. A study comparing medically led care with birth in Third World countries without medical backup will have very different outcomes to a study comparing natural births with Caesarians in the First World with optimal care given in both cases.

The studies comparing Caesarean birth to vaginal birth show that with a Caesarean delivery:
- Women spend three times as long in hospital [50]
- They are four times as likely to suffer from an infection [51]
- They are five times as likely to have an emergency hysterectomy [52]
- They are five times as likely to be readmitted to hospital with complications after they have been discharged [53]
- They are two to five times more likely to die giving birth [54]
- They have ten times the need for narcotic pain relief [55]
- They have two and a half times poorer birth experiences [56]
- They have less early contact with their babies to initiate bonding and are less likely to initiate play with their babies in the first five months postpartum. [57]

Babies who have been delivered by Caesarean:
- Are four times as likely to die at birth, and when these statistics have been adjusted for potential confounding variables, they still have double the risk of dying. [58, 59] An important cause of infant death is respiratory distress syndrome, which is much higher in babies born by Caesarean birth. This is partly because these infants are sometimes mistakenly delivered prematurely and partly due to the fact that their lungs are still filled with fluid after a Caesarean and, therefore, the adjustment to extra uterine breathing is more difficult for these babies. The lack of birthing hormones present in the baby's body may add to the likelihood of her developing respiratory distress syndrome. Adjustment to extra uterine breathing may also be impeded by the umbilical cord being cut immediately, creating no transition time for babies to adjust to receiving oxygen through their lungs rather than from the placenta

- Are four times as likely to have dangerously low Apgar scores of 0–3 at five minutes [60]
- Are less likely to be breastfed and are twice as likely to have breastfeeding difficulties. [61]

Long-term problems include the perceived need for subsequent Caesareans.
- The risk of delivery increases exponentially as the number of previous Caesareans increases. This is mostly due to an increased risk of placenta previa and placenta accreta [62, 63, 64]
- A 20 percent increase in the likelihood of the child developing diabetes mellitus, according to a recently published meta analysis. [65]

Many women are told that urinary incontinence is such a problem after a vaginal delivery that it is worth having a Caesarean to avoid future problems.
- While there is an increased risk of urinary incontinence in women who have given birth vaginally, Dr Sakala looked at all the studies on post-birth urinary incontinence that had been done up to 2006, comparing vaginal birth to Caesarean, and none of them "attempted to minimize or control for harmful co-interventions" [66] when considering whether giving birth through the vagina increased the risk of pelvic floor problems. However, there is no doubt that pelvic floor injury is increased by:
- Cutting an episiotomy
- Vacuum- and forceps-assisted deliveries
- Lying on your back to give birth
- Encouragement of strained pushing to get your baby out, rather than encouraging you to relax your pelvic outlet during the pushing phase
- Pressing on your abdomen to force your baby out.

Why then are Caesareans sold to us as being easier, safer, and less damaging to our bodies, when clearly these are obstetrical myths? In the South African private sector during the last ten years, the rate of Caesarean deliveries has risen from 30 percent to more than 70 percent. Possible reasons for the rising rate of Caesarean births have been attributed to the following causative factors:
- Health insurance companies pay out for Caesareans without requiring a medical necessity
- The art of normal delivery is being lost as obstetricians spend more time in the operating theater than in delivery rooms
- We are developing casual attitudes about surgery, even though a Caesarean is still a major abdominal operation

- We are being taught to fear natural birth: too often we are told that our "baby is too big," when often they may be of average size. Big babies birth just fine with a little bit of patience, especially when we are encouraged to birth in the positions of our choice rather than having to lie flat on our backs
- Caesarean birth is a common "side effect" of medical procedures such as induction or episiotomies
- There is too little time and care and support given to women in labor. As such, we midwives are failing to support normal physiological labor
- Convenience is a big factor for choosing elective Caesareans, both among women and their caregivers
- Caesarean birth rates increase dramatically in countries where there is no policy supporting a trial of labor for women who have had a previous Caesarean. The "Once a Caesarean, always a Caesarean" policy is outdated
- Normal births attended by obstetricians rather than by midwives increase the likelihood of Caesarean births [67]
- I hesitate to quote the following factor as a cause of rising Caesarean birth rates, as the obstetricians I know personally are genuinely caring individuals, who truly have their patients' best interests at heart. However, in South Africa, private obstetricians, who do the most Caesarean births, get paid more for performing them than they do for vaginal births
- Women may choose a Caeseran birth out of fear of natural birth.

Absolute indications for a Caesarean birth include:
- Cord prolapse
- Maternal pelvic contraction, such as that caused by rickets, malformations, or injury to the pelvis
- Hemorrhagic conditions, e.g. complete placenta previa or placental abruption
- Transverse presentation that refuses to budge.

Caesarean births, even inevitable ones that do not happen out of choice, can be controled to a certain extent by the mother. It is possible to request certain approaches to the management of the operation. It is possible to choose an obstetrician who respects our requests, even if they decide in consultation with us that they do not feel comfortable honoring all our requests. We have options for creating conditions for Caesareans that are supportive and gentle for our babies.

Zann Hoad had her third baby by elective Caesarean in Johannesburg. Having accepted that this was the safest method for her to birth her baby she researched all the ways she felt she could improve the experience for the baby. She called this a "natural Caesarean." She found a hospital in the United Kingdom where staff advised her that the most important factors to help her baby adjust to extra uterine life were:

- To go into labor naturally, so that the baby was ready for birth and her labor hormones had crossed her placenta into her baby's body, rather than have a date scheduled beforehand;
- To dim the operating theater lights;
- To warm up the operating theater when she first went into labor, since they are routinely kept very cold to minimize infection;
- To have the baby placed immediately on her chest skin to skin and covered with a pre-warmed towel. Hospital gowns and sterile fields may make skin-to-skin contact difficult for some theaters to allow—even though this is the best way for her baby to maintain their thermal equilibrium. Wrapping the baby in a warm towel and placing him on your chest is a less effective but acceptable alternative;
- To leave the umbilical cord uncut for thirty seconds, with her baby placed lower than her abdomen—perhaps between her legs, to allow for an effective placental transfusion of blood through to her baby. The blood provides oxygen in the first moments after birth and also supplies him with extra iron in the months following birth. A thirty-second delay in umbilical cord clamping will also allow the fluid to begin to clear from his lungs before he takes his first breath. (See umbilical cord clamping page 193–197.) Even though your obstetrician may be hesitant to delay the process of closing your uterine wound while waiting for blood transfer to occur from your placenta to your baby after delivery, it is a procedure that is becoming standard practice in some hospitals in the United Kingdom. It is undoubtedly less traumatic for your baby to be given this short time to learn how to breathe before having to breathe in order to survive. Delayed cutting of the umbilical cord, however, needs to be weighed up against immediate placement of your baby skin to skin on your chest;
- To have the pediatrician check the baby on her chest rather than on the resuscitation table where they are normally checked;
- For the short while that her baby is separated from her, to have him kangarooed skin to skin by her husband or held in a warm basin of water.

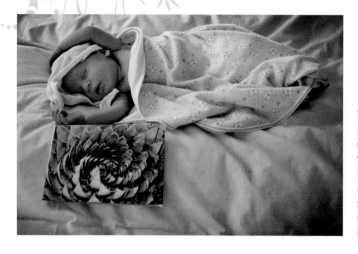

Vince, with a photo of an aloe, spiraling like a thousand-petaled lotus, which represented the spiral of giving and receiving to Zann in a dream.

Zann's Caesarean births

I ended up having Caesarean births for all my children. Until recently I felt sad about this. My fantasy was always to have that "empowered" natural birth. I think sometimes the mythology of our childhoods end up scripting our stories in adult life. I was always told that my hips were very narrow—somehow, deep down I didn't believe that my body was up for the challenge.

Max's birth, 1997

Even though it was a hospital environment, I was planning to have a water birth with midwives at Bedford clinic. When I arrived they gave me an enema. I was a bit surprised. I expected the midwives to be more caring. They were just like paramedics; they didn't know of the mind-body connection or, if they did, they didn't feel confident in expressing it. I had thought I was managing fine with the contractions, but eventually the midwives offered me pethidine, and after the injection I gave up, I felt like I gave away my power.

After that I didn't dilate properly. It was a long, arduous labor. I labored through the night with a terrible gynecologist. I was lying on my back with my legs in stirrups, pushing. If I hadn't been on my back and feeling so powerless, it might have been different. I pushed for three hours, but Max wouldn't budge. They tried the vacuum three times, and he wouldn't come out. Fred and the gynecologist were standing be-

tween my legs discussing the problem, like a business meeting—what they should do. I yelled at them to stop talking as if it was an arbitrary event. So they did an emergency Caesarean.

I suppose I feel a kind of anger at myself for not knowing it could have been different. If only I'd known what I know now. I hold a sadness that that's what women are subjected to, because they don't know better. It's iniquitous, unnecessary, and like we're being robbed, in a way. It's so subtle, because just being in a hospital is the wrong place, and it's so easy for women to feel intimidated there. We're shy about our bodies, our nakedness. We feel exposed, and then we can't do the work of birth with the same centeredness.

We have to feel safe to birth. I'd thought birth was such a primal thing that it would override what was happening around me. But so much of what your mind is saying to your body influences birth. I remember feeling so afraid of shitting myself.

Being supported and loved and cared for by my midwives could have changed the quality of my labor. In labor, I felt so vulnerable and out of my normal self. I chose midwives to support me in labor because doctors are trained to work from an intellectual head space, where they have an unconscious assumption that I am a patient with a medical emergency and they are going to solve it.

I think most people haven't had an experience of deep meditation and of feeling their central core of power. If I'd had that experience in my life before I labored with Max, if I could have drawn on that deep powerful center in myself, I'm sure that would have helped me. But I didn't know that then.

Despite all that, Max and I were perfectly connected. He was a sweet, loving, loved baby. It was a very happy time. The horrible experience paled quite quickly. I was disappointed, but I was okay. He did have a red, puffy bruise on his head. He's eleven now and still has a raised ridge there. As a child these days, he's very centered and still, but quite reticent, also—he doesn't make friends very easily. Other kids are attracted to him, though. He has a quiet confidence, and he's quite interesting—like he has suffered, but he has processed it. He has a natural emotional intelligence. A graceful way of resolving conflict… a deeply warm, empathetic person.

The centeredness we can draw on in labor reminds me of when we were hijacked in the driveway; almost instinctively, intuitively, I went into that deep, quiet center in myself. Consequently, I was not traumatized at the time. The whole thing was calm, and I felt very protected. I think in labor if you can go there, that's the place that channels >

the universal life stream. I have a deep sense that there's a truth there. Visually, inside myself, I see a cylinder shape in my body that is filled with universal love and light, it extends up through my neck and head and pours in there. I hold it in myself, in my consciousness. I suppose its defining quality is that it's utterly still and connects with everything around me. And also in a way, in that space, there's no good and no bad. So in the hijacking, it was just an event—these people wanted to take our stuff, and we gave it to them. In labor, if you can get past the fear of what your body is doing, then it can be so beautiful. Then there is no good or bad—that's the essence of it.

Jet's birth, 1998

Jetty was rushed at birth, and I think perhaps it's had lifelong consequences for her. She was born fifteen months after Max. The midwives and the doctors all said that the scar was too new and I couldn't risk a labor in case of uterine rupture. I trusted that that was right. However, even though they said she was full term, I think she was two weeks premature. She weighed 3.3 kilograms (7.3 pounds), but she was covered in vernix, and emotionally she wasn't ready, we had done no preparation.

Before she was born by elective Caesarean, I didn't talk to her. I didn't tell her about being born; I didn't know you could. So she had no idea. I went to hospital with my lipstick and eyeliner on. Fred met me there. It was very clinical. She was born with bright lights, in a cold theater, and I was a bit disengaged. I think she was a bit stuck; they yanked her out by her foot. In a subsequent hypnotherapy process I re-experienced my own birth, being pulled out by one foot, too, and they all laughed at me (the doctors said I looked like a naked chicken). Jet's birth mirrored my birth, and the two of us have a deep connection.

In theater, as soon as the baby is out, she goes to the pediatrician, and the doctor lets go of his responsibility for the baby. This is a transitional zone the baby is in. I'd like to hazard a wild guess here about Jet's birth. Her cord was cut instantly, and she struggles now in changing of activities; she fights change. We call it "Transitional Anxiety." Like a trapeze artist, letting go of one swinging bar and flying through the air to catch the other one, that gap in the changing of activities causes a lot of children these days a lot of anxiety. Maybe it's because that transition between breathing with the umbilical cord and breathing air is so swift these days. Nowadays, the supply from the umbilical cord is chopped off immediately, and perhaps this causes children to experience huge transitional anxiety, as they haven't been given enough time to absorb the fluid that is filling their lungs at birth. So they are left literally gasping for breath.

In hospital, after the birth, Jet wouldn't let me put her down. She wouldn't sleep in her crib; she cried there. She would only sleep in the crook of my arm. It's as though the way she feels love in the world is through physical touch—she really needs and wants it. She likes to kiss and hug and cuddle all the time, even though most girls of nine don't like to do that.

Jet is speedy, swift, and noisy. She bounces off the walls, and sometimes it feels as if she's rattling at a million miles an hour. Sometimes I have to ask her to breathe and slow down. Her life experience so far is offering her incredible opportunities for personal development, but it's hard. Her health has always been very fragile, and in a funny way, I think she needs all this grist for her mill. She's an amazing musician and artist, and maybe she needed that birth to give her material. However, I can see that even though on the one hand we choose everything in our lives at a deep mystical level, we do need to make conscious choices about how we give birth. As human beings we have an ethical, moral, humane capacity to reach out to create conditions that support others.

Jet is an extraordinary child—highly strung, high maintenance. She has huge potential as a creative force in the world. It's really beautiful and exciting to recognize the multi-layered connectedness of all these things, to learn to connect and discover all the tissue paper layers. It's so rewarding. Jet is an amazing individual. It's quite a journey.

If I understand emotionally and intellectually what's happening in my births, I'm so much more empowered to read my children. Since Jet's birth, I've been able to identify the link between what happened during her birth and her emotional side. If I didn't recognize that link I'd find it really difficult. If I come to understand what happened and go there in a non-judgmental way, it helps me to be a better parent. If I unpack what really happened, unconditionally, I can understand my child.

Vince's birth, 2006

I consciously accessed that still, centered place for Vince's birth. I played the whistling song—"Love Generation"—in the operating theater. I'd been playing it all through pregnancy. I felt connected with Vince, and I also spoke to him: "You know you're going to be born; this is our song." I also went into labor with Vinnie, even though the doctor was adamant that that was more dangerous because it might >

mean an emergency Caesarean. I went into labor at four in the morning, Vince was eventually born by Caesarean at 6 p.m., and I knew that he was ready to come out. I'd done hypnotherapy and met Vince during the session a month before. He told me "I'm going to be born on the 20th." His due date was the 26th. I'd negotiated with the doctor that if he was not born by the 26th, then he could do the Caesarean. Vince knew all along. He said, "Don't worry about the actual date, I'm coming on the 20th." Afterward, the gynecologist said to me, "I told you so. We should have done the Caesarean before his due date"!

When I fell pregnant with Vince, I wanted to try for a natural birth. I had done lots of spiritual work in the previous ten years. I phoned a number of doctors. There was only one doctor who would allow me to attempt a vaginal birth after two previous Caesareans. But he lived in the Eastern Cape, and it wasn't feasible for me to move there for the birth. So I found an independent midwife who agreed to accompany me to the Caesarean, and she recommended a progressive obstetrician who was interested in natural birth. It took a lot to persuade him around my medical needs. I wrote him a letter eventually, at my last visit before Vince was born. He was quite resistant, but he did agree to most of the points.

Women need to be prepared that this is not an easy negotiation. It has to be done with charm and persistence, not a fight. Medical professionals can be resistant. I said, I respect your knowledge, but there are some things that are important to me. I took that kind of approach. If your obstetrician says "no" then try again and again.

It's hard because we are disempowered in that situation, anyway. No way can we do the negotiations in theater; it all has to be negotiated beforehand. Women need to be prepared for a long, hard negotiation because that is what it takes. It's worth fighting a bit harder for the most important things.

Almost everything on my list, my doctor agreed to, though. I looked at photos yesterday on the computer, and there was one photo of Vince as he was taken out of my body—he was on the operating table between my legs. I thought he was put straight on my chest. Even though there was a tiny bit of medical intervention, which was necessary because he had meconium in his amniotic fluid, so they needed to suction him, it still felt good. I think he was aware of our intentions and that was important.

The operating staff created the usual sterile field from below my breasts rather than above them, and they put the electrodes on my sides instead of on my chest. So that as soon as they had suctioned him, they could put him skin to skin on my chest.

He was a sticky little bundle coming onto my chest. He latched then. It was wonderful to see my newborn on my breast; there was such power in his will to live, a raw, survival energy that comes from that. It's magnificent. It seems like such an arbitrary thing, but it's not. Jet was taken away from me after her birth, and when they wheeled me to the room, I didn't know where she was. Vince never, ever left me, even when they sewed me up. He was placed in warm water in a little tub next to me, with his dad holding him.

I needed to have an independent midwife with me to ensure that all my requests were honored. Someone I trusted and who I knew would do what I wanted, who put a hat on him and a warm towel so that he could remain skin to skin on my chest without getting cold. She said, "Don't wipe him down and wrap him up." The medical staff in the theater won't do all that. Then she put him in the water. But she knew not to interfere with the pediatrician. I paid for a consultation with the pediatrician prior to the birth, so that we could agree on my special requests. Vince was checked by her while he was on my body.

Vince was very calm, very quiet; he didn't even cry. He just looked into our eyes, intense and very sweet, beautiful, healing. I had a bizarre experience a day later. He was looking into my eyes, and it felt like my body and consciousness were catapulted through time and space, as if I were traveling at an incredible speed into a space of peace and love. Like a sci-fi movie of being shot out into space. And he was holding me as I went through that.

When Vince was a week old, I had an incredible dream. Pritam, my yoga teacher said to me in the dream, "Life is a continuous giving and receiving, like the spiraling of a thousand-petal lotus." That same day, I found a picture in a magazine of an aloe, growing in spirals, like a thousand-petal lotus. I have a photo of Vince next to the aloe—that was the intuitive message he was giving me.

Now he's bigger—twenty-one months. The other day I was driving, and I looked back in the rearview mirror and said, "Vince, you're a beautiful boy." And he said, "Momma, beautiful boy." I'm his "beautiful boy," too. He has quite a sophisticated emotional repertoire. I'm sure it's because of who he is as a person, but also because of how he's been handled. I feel a deep sense of respect for him. He naturally requires that we listen carefully to his needs. His communication is very clear. And consequently, he cries very little. It feels like an equal relationship, where the power is in balance. We are not so much parenting him as listening to him show us the way.

No matter the choices we make, birth, like the babies we produce, has its own agenda and follows its own path, which may not fit in with our plans and expectations. Mothers who take a stand and make informed choices for their birth places and attendants, while letting go of any expectations for the unfolding of the birth, are the ones whose bonding with their babies is statistically the most favorable.

Provided everybody is well and healthy, it is as much how we approach the birth and parenting as how they unfold that seems to create the most positive emotional outcomes for the family. Love flows through the breast milk and nourishes the baby more than the milk itself; however, love can flow through bottled milk, too. In spite of circumstances, if the love is there, it will find its way to a baby through a plastic teat from a doped up and exhausted mother in a disruptive ward with bossy nurses and unhelpful schedules.

Choice of caregiver

> The thing that helps more than anything (at a birth) is that the person who's helping you loves you. It can make the difference between heavy complications and having a nice time.
>
> — Ina May Gaskin, American midwife, author of Spiritual Midwifery [68]

One of the most important decisions to be made for labor is your choice of midwife or obstetrician. The impact they will have on the atmosphere in the birthing room is enormous. Women who have spent months preparing for birth with relaxation techniques can find the going gets tough if they have no one other than their husband supporting them emotionally during labor. If you would like to experience labor and natural birth you should find a caregiver who has real trust that your body knows how to labor and that, given a calm secure environment, you will do just fine. Interview your potential caregivers before you make your birth choice—speak to obstetricians, midwives in private practice, and midwives in labor wards. You should not only feel relaxed and comfortable with them as people, you should also ensure that their protocols for birthing match your ideas about how you would like to give birth.

If you want an elective Caesarean, choose an obstetrician who is well recommended for their sensitive management of the operating room atmosphere and surgical skills, as well as for how quickly their scars heal. You should still feel comfortable with them as people, and they should still give you as much time as you need during antenatal consultations. Most importantly, they should be flexible enough in their surgical approach to acknowledge that this is your birth and that your choices for the birth atmosphere should be honored and respected as much as possible.

If you want a natural birth, choose a few questions from the list below that you feel are important to you in order to get an idea of your potential caregiver's approach to birth. Asking all of them might be stretching their patience at a single interview:

- How much time will you be with me in labor and after the birth?
- Who else will be monitoring me if you're not there, and will I get to meet them beforehand?
- What would your reasons be for deciding to induce me?
- What would your reasons be for deciding to deliver my baby by Caesarean birth?
- What do you think of natural birth? How would you support me best if I choose to experience natural birth without pain relief? I have heard that epidural labors often require vacuum or forceps assistance for birth. What is your response to that?
- How many of your clients have Caesareans? Some obstetricians have a Caesarean birth rate of more than 70 percent. According to the World Health Organisation (WHO), Caesarean rates of more than 7–10 percent are not beneficial for mother or baby.
- How long will you allow my baby to remain in my uterus past my due date?
- Will you induce if my baby is "too big?"
- How long will you allow before inducing labor after my waters have broken?
- Will you leave the umbilical cord uncut until it has stopped pulsating?
- How will you support me emotionally during my labor, or how would you suggest I create an atmosphere of emotional support during labor?
- How important do you think the atmosphere in the birth room is?
- May I adopt any position for giving birth in or do you require me to lie on my back?
- Do you deliver babies underwater?

How your caregiver responds to your questions is more important than which questions you ask. Be aware of the quality of their attention. You are looking for someone who will ensure that not only are you and your baby safe and physically well but also that you are emotionally supported. Notice if they:

- Like people

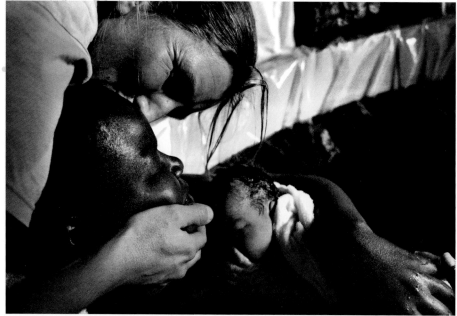

Choose a caregiver whom you relate to well and who will support your birth choices.

- Trust natural birth
- Trust that your body knows how to birth
- Are relaxed and easygoing
- Are tender and compassionate
- Are concerned for you emotional and physical well-being
- Are patient and unrushed—both in themselves and in their attitude toward you
- Are comfortable in their own bodies. If they are not, will they trust yours to know what to do?
- Finally, labor is intimate, so ask yourself if you are comfortable with them touching you.

 To thine own self be true, and it must follow, as the night the day, thou canst not then be false to any man.

— *William Shakespeare* [69]

Midwives

> In the hospital, I hadn't perceived the anxiety and foreboding that permeated birth until I experienced the impact of its absence among the midwives. The peace, wonder, and intimacy were infinitely greater. What a compelling difference!

— *Heidi Rinehart, MD* [70]

The way we perceive our experience of birth does depend on how we are treated as laboring women. If we are encouraged to trust that this birth belongs to us and to our babies, not to our caregivers and the hospitals, then we have the opportunity to truly transform and to give birth to the responsible mother within us. Midwives, if they are the primary caregivers, often believe in birth's ability to empower women, and so they are more likely to encourage them to listen to their bodies in labor.

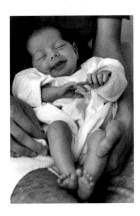

Sue's first born, Rebecca, smiling within days of her birth.

Sue Lees

Sue Lees is a wonderful midwife in Cape Town—she was the primary caregiver for many of the women whose stories about birth enrich this book. Sue has this to say about her approach to midwifery:

Easy, magnificent births happen when women acknowledge what a rite of passage the birth process is, and when we midwives acknowledge the rite of passage. As caregivers, we can let birth become very routine, so it's important to stop and remember that this is an enormous event taking place.

>

The mothers can sometimes do a lot in terms of preparation and clearing obstacles, fears, and prejudices, but it helps them to acknowledge that birth unfolds in its own way, not necessarily the way they might want it to.

Because we midwives live in the world, with peripheral lives, families, and worldly irritations, I often find myself in a tired or irritable place when I am called to a birth. On the way to the labor I have to acknowledge that now is the time to put peripheral concerns aside. The mother will only experience birth a couple of times in her life. The experience she has will impact on how she conducts herself as a woman in the world for the rest of her life. It's so connected to her self-esteem.

So from a personal point of view, I make a conscious effort to put my attitudes and feelings aside, to be as present as I can for that woman at that time. Afterward, she will view herself based on how the birth was for her, which is also dependent on how it was facilitated. The outcome of the birth, whether she has a Caesarean or a vaginal birth, is not so important. What is important is how each aspect of the birth is honored. It is important to allow the mother to honor that it isn't just her process but the baby's, too. It is possible for her to have a satisfying outcome, even if the birth isn't as she envisaged.

I was at a birth recently where Kathy dilated only two centimeters (0.79 inches) between 10.30 a.m. and 8.30 p.m. I was aware that it was immaterial what I suggested if she wasn't ready for it yet. It was important just to honor the process she needed to go through. She eventually had a Caesarean at 10 p.m. Giving my professional opinion, and then allowing them to come to their own decisions in their own time, helped them to leave the birth process satisfied that it was their process, so that although they were sad they had a Caesarean, there was an understanding and an acceptance. They didn't feel manipulated by somebody's language of fear into doing things they were not ready to do. If mothers can feel that they are making the decisions, they can move into mothering feeling like it was their birth. The caregiver moves on to the next birth, but that mother is left with her experience.

BIRTH PREPARATION

Chapter Four

> "You hear a slogan like 'Always maintain only a joyful mind,' and for the whole next two weeks you're just hitting yourself over the head for never being joyful. That kind of witness is a bit heavy. So lighten up. Don't make such a big deal. The key to feeling at home with your body, mind, and emotions, to feeling worthy to live on this planet, comes from being able to lighten up. This earnestness, this seriousness about everything in our lives—including practice—this goal-oriented, 'we're going to do it or else' attitude, is the world's greatest killjoy. There's no sense of appreciation because we're so solemn about everything. In contrast, a joyful mind is very ordinary and relaxed."
>
> — *Pema Chödrön, Author and Buddhist nun in Tibetan tradition* [71]

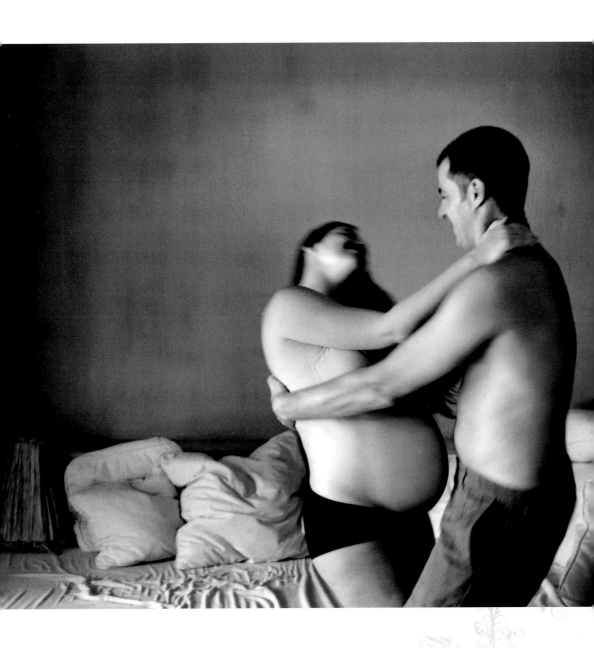

When considering which techniques to choose for labor, ask yourself if they will help you to respond to labor in a flexible, easy way. Labor is the domain of the feminine. Don't think of the feminine as weak, modest, and submissive. An empowered female embodies qualities of gracious receptivity, a nurturing open heart, and an ability to flow with each present moment. Labor techniques are helpful if they create conditions for responding intuitively to your body and your baby. Responses do not exclude making a noise and expressing powerfully strong energy.

So, in choosing birth preparation techniques, look for ones that will help you develop awareness—awareness of all levels of consciousness, awareness of your baby and of yourself. And look for techniques that increase the atmosphere of love and support in the birthing room, for yourself, for your baby and for your partner. Bringing a spacious, open heart to labor opens your cervix and tells your baby that this is a safe and welcoming world. It conveys an impression of trust, which is the sense that is going to help her to easily move out of your womb and into life.

There are many hundreds of effective methods of preparing for birth, most of which can be tremendously helpful. Physical preparation includes excellent nutrition and myriad forms of exercise to tone the body and increase flexibility and pelvic movement. Mental preparation includes training our minds to focus and to relax into the process of birth. Emotional preparation can deal with releasing any fears we have around the labor and birth that could impact negatively on the natural unfolding of the birth, and spiritual preparation includes connecting with our babies on a soul level, on developing our ability to stay centered, and on creating an atmosphere of love and support in the birth room with which to nurture ourselves and our babies.

Birth preparation ideas

- Learning techniques for letting go of rigidity and resistance
- Communicating with your unborn child to find out her needs for birth and for remaining aware of your connection during labor
- Connecting with your partner and having them be fully there for you emotionally
- Ensuring that your labor support team includes someone who has a deep understanding of birth and is experienced in encouraging women to feel safe during labor

- Choosing caregivers who will make any medical or birth decisions in full consultation with you and who respect that their participation in the birth is as a support person rather than as the person in charge of the process
- Becoming informed about birth and parenting choices
- Meditation for letting go into each moment anew
- Visualization to encourage your cervix to open easily
- Toning to create a sense of harmonic resonance in your body
- Dance for intimacy and settling into the limbic brain
- Deep relaxation techniques and guided relaxation for birth
- Integration therapy to release old patterns of behavior that may impact on birthing and parenting
- Birth art for recognizing what your unconscious expectations of the birth are
- Belly-casts for remembering how beautiful your body became in pregnancy
- Enjoying your pregnant body and looking after it with good nutrition and beneficial exercise
- Birth ceremonies for acknowledging your transition into motherhood
- Setting up a birth pool wherever you plan to give birth.

Be gentle with yourself

Pregnancy can be emotionally and physically challenging. It is not easy to share our bodies with a little person for forty weeks. So often we are led to believe that pregnancy is so normal that we should almost ignore it and simply carry on with life. Some women need to nurture themselves with extra care and love during pregnancy.

- Take time out
- Nap
- Sit in the sun
- Enjoy a cup of tea with a friend
- Breathe happiness down into your body, and occasionally breathe out a huge sigh of relief—the kind of relief that says, "Phew! I got here. Right here, into this very moment. Finally, I arrived! How wonderful."

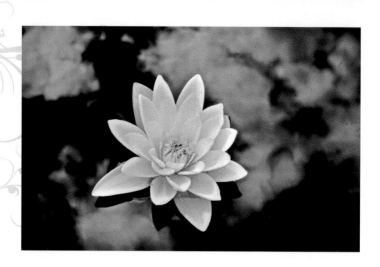

Meditation

" Develop a mind that is vast like the water. Where experience, both pleasant and unpleasant, can appear or disappear without conflict, struggle, or harm. Rest in a mind that is vast like the water. "

— *Gautama Buddha, founder of Buddhism, 4th century BCE*

Meditation is simple in concept. It is the art of listening, of awareness, of mindfulness in the present moment. We have a tendency to complicate it in application. We are sometimes loath to subject the little dramas of our lives to the scrutiny of meditation or we think that the purpose of meditation is to become peaceful, perfect, and enlightened. Not so. Even though the subject of meditation is vast enough to fill volumes, the purpose of meditation is to simply be with what is.

Meditation is not a quick-fix technique. It slowly and patiently teaches us objectivity— the ability to see another person's point of view when we are caught in emotional entrapment. It teaches us to smile at our inconsistencies and our irrational manipulations. Meditation, properly applied, can bring a heartful awareness to living.

When we meditate well we begin to notice the preciousness in life. We slow down enough to be aware of the wind rustling the branches of the tree around which two squirrels are chasing one another, to notice the potted plant that hasn't been watered, the elbow we bumped and hurt yesterday that requires more sympathy. We become more aware of our own hearts, sometimes small, sometimes sad, and the hearts of others—the underdressed man selling wire-beaded sunflowers in the rain, or our child with her perpetual "why"?

> 66 Still—in a way—nobody sees a flower;
> Really it is so small—we haven't time,
> And to see takes time,
> Like to have a friend takes time. 99
> — *Georgia O'Keeffe, American artist 1887 – 1986* [72]

Meditation is the art of attending to the small and the unnoticed. Mindfulness is the cornerstone of meditation activity. Mindfulness, used appropriately, develops compassion and opens the heart. Clarity and mindfulness develop from conscious awareness of what is happening in the present moment. To develop awareness, the focus of attention may be placed on the breath, on bodily sensations, sounds, a mantra, one's thoughts, on a Zen koan, on a visualization. The techniques are many, but they are like different paths up the same mountain.

We usually get farther up the path if we stick to one route for a while than if we come back down to try another and another. Nevertheless, dallying and obstacles occur frequently on this journey, so detours and scenic routes are an important part of it; if you stop to smell the flowers, you may come to the realization that that is the whole point of meditation—the flowers on the top of the mountain are no different, after all, than those on the way up.

Each second we settle into the equanimity of allowing this moment of awareness to simply be as it is, we do so not only for ourselves but for everybody around us as well. Change happens from within, one precious breath at a time. Thich Nhat Hanh, a beautiful Zen Master renowned for his simplicity and compassion, has many "gathas" or poems, like the following one for bringing attention into each moment:

> 66 Breathing in, I calm my body,
> Breathing out, I smile,
> Dwelling in the present moment,
> I know this is a wonderful moment. 99
> — *Thich Nhat Hanh, Zen master and peace activist* [73]

As we practice this simple meditation over and over, our breathing slows and deepens, our racing minds decelerate a little, and distracting thoughts move from center stage to the periphery of our consciousness. Babies are often the first to pick up on the more peaceful energy. As we practice settling more, we often begin to notice that people are more likely

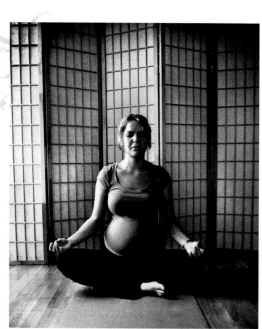

Meditation is the art of simply staying present in this moment.

to smile at us in the streets, even if we haven't acknowledged them first. Slowly, impercep-tibly, our world begins to change, to soften, to flower. Then, when challenges arise, we find there is space enough in our hearts to meet them openly and without avoidance.

If we must have a marker for meditation progress, we can best judge how we are doing by noticing if our hearts are becoming more open. Jack Kornfield, a Buddhist psychothera-pist, suggests we continuously ask ourselves whether this path has a heart. This approach can keep our meditation direction clear. As the Dalai Lama says, "My religion is kindness." Or in the words of Antoine de Saint-Exupery, "It is only with the heart that one can see rightly; what is essential is invisible to the eye."[74]

A young woman sitting under thatch eaves on a small wooden platform soon after she began practicing meditation became aware of the deeper essence beneath ordinary experi-ence, and was amazed to discover that it was identical to love. She didn't tell anybody, for fear of sounding evangelical, and she forgot it often in the years after the experience. But gradually it began to seep into her life in such a way that it permeated her consciousness, and nowadays it molds and shapes her experience of life. She says, "It took fifteen years to recognize how this was all I needed to know all along. Many workshops and meditation retreats later, the experience has deepened and settled within me; it has become some-thing I refer back to and use in everyday life."

To know how to make life choices wisely is to learn to become more aware of the sensitivity and nudges of intuitive feeling. This is nothing more nor less than stopping and notic-ing the myriad layers of what we are really feeling deep inside our bodies. Often we make our choices out of ambition or fear, both of which are states of mind that allow us to avoid how things really are in our life.

Meditation is the art of listening clearly and carefully until the spaciousness that devel-ops gives us more objective insights into the essence of our problems, concepts, and beliefs. We gradually move through the chaos and confusion of emotional entanglements, of want-ing and avoiding, to a state of awareness, objective vision, intuition, and seeing through the illusions. As we become more adept at meditation and more open, our sense of the world expands beyond a purely material reality. Our sense of having a separate self softens or melts and we become aware of the interdependence of all things.

We are all essentially enlightened, clear, calm, wise and light-filled, but we cloud our vision with our wants and needs, our likes and dislikes. In trying to control our world and have things go our way, in getting caught up in our narrow viewpoints, we block ourselves off from our clear, spacious, and very wise essence, which is who we truly are.

It's easy to develop equanimity, awareness, and clarity for moments at a time; a master remains so even in the face of death. We meditate in order to be able to remain open to all our experiences even when confronted with upheavals in our lives. Allowing life to unfold without resistance doesn't mean not changing the things that need to be changed, or not standing up for what you believe is right; it means seeing each situation clearly, without the emotional clouding of anger, fear, and sadness. This is an interesting concept, because it doesn't mean not feeling anger, fear, or sadness. Emotions are as they are, and are part of our human condition. Identifying those emotions as belonging to us, and judging them as good or bad, is where the clouding arises.

If we ignore and suppress our feelings we live our lives half alive, half asleep, which is where most of us are a good deal of the time. If we express all our negative feelings as and when they wish to burst out of us, we create havoc and hurt and confusion.

All we need to do is simply bring awareness to every situation, to every feeling, and see where it affects our physical body, with the most scrupulous attention and without judging. Then, like a child demanding attention by pulling at our sleeves and happily disappearing as soon as we give her what she needs, the negativity is released through our attention.

We can't stop the waves, but we can learn to surf them. Meditation is neither shutting things off nor out. It helps us to see things more clearly, and to deliberately position our-selves differently in relationship to them.

How to meditate

> The mind of a holy person is like a mirror,
> Which neither grasps nor resists;
> It receives and lets go.
> That is why the sage encompasses
> The world without hurt. "
>
> — *Chuang-tzu, Taoist philosopher, 4th century BCE*

The meditations suggested here are ways to begin developing awareness. Often meditators find it helpful to have somebody who has walked this path before them to give them some direct guidance on their process. Receiving objective feedback about our meditation from someone who has an experiential understanding of the meditative process can help us avoid many hours of floundering and not being too sure of what is going on.

I meditate best if I bring some enjoyment to the process, otherwise I won't do it for long. I meditate as a restful exploration, as a gift to myself. Start with between five and twenty minutes a day. This is much less difficult than setting up a punishing schedule from the outset. Regularity is more beneficial than quantity, and it is better to spend five minutes with focused attention than twenty minutes dreaming.

Try meditating with the spine straight and upright, in as comfortable a position as is manageable. Cross-legged may be comfortable for longer periods of time, which is why it is the conventional meditation posture; however, it may be difficult to get used to initially. It is also okay to sit on a chair without leaning against the back of it, feet planted on the ground, and spine straight.

Lying down, unless I'm listening to a guided visualization or practicing deep relaxation, is often so restful that I fall asleep. Subtle life-force energy moves more freely though a vertical spinal column than a horizontal one. Some Tibetan meditation practitioners may spend months or years at a time never allowing their bodies to move farther than forty-five degrees from the vertical plane in order to maintain a clear pranic flow of energy—these guys even sleep sitting up!

It's useful to always adopt the same posture. My body quickly learns to become centered and focused in meditation posture as soon as I assume it. Breathing is important. It's a focus for my attention, and it's always there. It is also our major source of prana, the subtle life-force energy. Breathing deeply helps me to relax, center, and focus my mind. The whole system of body, mind, and spirit is involved. Meditate without having expectations, without judging, without expecting special states of being, without needing to be good at it. Some-

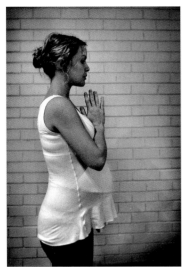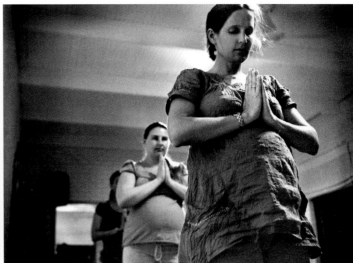

Letting go into the simplicity of being here, now.

times the most beneficial meditation might be one of intense boredom and staying open to that state of mind. I can learn more about myself through difficult meditation experiences than through accessing altered states of consciousness and light-filled heavenly realms. Light realms are wonderful to experience, so long as I can allow that they aren't permanent at my level of development and that they aren't a measure of how good I am at meditating.

Meditate walking, running, taking a bath. It simply requires intentionality. Meditation is not necessarily a special state. It's about feeling the way I feel—simply sitting, breathing, watching, listening, and feeling what is. It involves:

- Making space for myself.
- Making space for even my fears to be just the way they are. By recognizing a fear and being open enough to it, I see beneath it to what it is in life that I am not able to trust. The easiest way to identify a fear is to recognize that a feeling is there, and then to name it as precisely as I can—by noticing where it is in my body, what sensations are being produced, and what my reaction is to those sensations.
- If I can do that, I can simply be with anger or fear or mistrust if it is there and make space for it.
- Letting go of likes and dislikes. Non-judging. I tend to judge even my meditation all the time.
- Intense awareness in a calm, clear, open, relaxed manner. Or, intense awareness in a bored, angry, or emotionally turbulent state of mind. Either is just okay.

Simplicity meditation

Breathing in. Breathing out. I bring awareness into my belly. Letting go into the simplicity of being here, now.

Just this much.

I feel the peace that arises from not needing to change anything in this moment. No judgment. No need to be perfect, better, or other than I am. Just breathing. Simple awareness of the inflow and the outflow of the breath.

Opening to the moment.

Developing awareness of the almost imperceptible, through noticing what is happening with the finest and most delicate observation.

Observing thoughts. Letting go. Allowing thoughts to pass by without getting caught up in them.

Observing pain. Letting go. Allowing things to be as they are.

Letting go into the moment. Allowing my mind and myself to be as I am.

Allowing any feelings that arise to be just the way they are with a simple acceptance of being in this moment. I sense how it feels in my body without resisting any sensations. Over and over until, with focused awareness, they begin to dissolve of their own accord.

Breath flowing in, breath ebbing away. In and out.

Feeling the breath in my belly.

My belly and my body does not know or judge. Belly simply experiences.

Feeling the peace and spaciousness that arises from experiencing life in this moment.

Trusting the way this moment is. I trust that it is safe to let go of past and future, of expectations and worries and judgments, to let go into breathing in and breathing out. I make space to experience life like a newborn child does. No preconceptions. Just simple experience. I trust that it is okay to be fully in each moment of experience.

I let go of needing things to be different from the way they already are, or of preferring an experience of bliss in meditation to one of boredom.

I let go of wanting this moment to be different,

And I settle into how it really is.

Feeling the peace there.

Breathing in, breath expands my belly. Breathing out, I let go into vast spaciousness.

Embracing awareness

" When we birth consciously, putting our great rational mind on hold and allowing our instinctive nature to dominate, we can access the wisdom that all spiritual traditions teach: the ego is our servant, not our mistress; and our path to ecstasy and enlightenment involves surrendering our egotistical notions of control. "

— *Dr. Sarah J. Buckley, Australian MD* [75]

Paying attention to any tension held in our bodies prior to birth can help us to recognize the sensations of rigidity and stress that may arise during labor and early parenting. Tension and stress during the newborn months may have been picked up from issues as diverse as the unease of our parents at our own births or the hectic schedule of our daily lives.

Resisting experiences and refusing to feel them fully means that we trap the energy relating to those experiences in the body. All emotions, when they are recognized in the body where we store them, will disappear and change, given full attention and an embracing awareness. The late Indian spiritual teacher Krishnamurti said that our attention allows emotions to "flower and fade." Letting them come to full fruition through simple awareness, they disappear of their own accord, and then we uncover a sense of greater spaciousness and ease. In this way, we soften the rigidity that has crept unnoticed into our bodies throughout our lives.

We need to hold a stable awareness in order to dissolve the holding patterns or to allow patterns to flower and fade. If attention is fragmented and unstable, holding patterns will not dissolve easily. The type of attention needed is not so much a focused concentration but a more spacious, gentle, and clear awareness. This process requires a certain amount of patience. Holding patterns can recur, even after they seem to disappear. Too much expectation of a quick fix could hamper the process, which requires a larger sense of infinite time, a timelessness.

So staying open to each emotion, be it fear, anger, or even heart-wrenching falling in love, over and over, is the key to it flowering freely and fading away of its own accord. This does not refer to acting on the feelings; it simply means paying bare attention and being fully present to the sensations created in the body without any resistance or reaction. This awareness changes our habitual patterns and releases them eventually. As Pema Chödrön

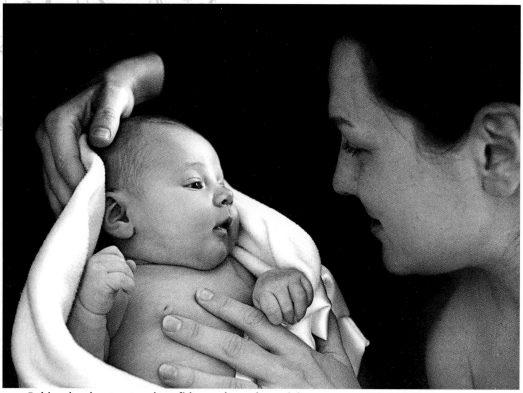

Babies develop trust and confidence through receiving unconditional acceptance and love.

says, "If your everyday practice is to open to all your emotions, to all the situations you encounter, without closing down, trusting that you can do that, then that will take you as far as you can go. And then you will understand all the teachings that anyone has ever taught."[76]

The tension we hold can impact our babies. In the first months after birth, baby-parent energy is so entwined that our anxiety at our inexperience, or our grumpiness as a result of being constantly woken, can be picked up and felt in our baby's body as his own anxiety or grumpiness.

Nisargadatta, a highly realized Hindu saint, refers to a sense of "I Amness" that is planted in the embryo in a dormant state. This sense seems to remain semidormant in young babies. They are aware of a sense of self, in that they cry if their body experiences pain and they gurgle when they are comforted; yet, they do not discriminate between their hand stroking their mother's breast as they feed, or the breast that is being stroked. Both are perceived as part of their consciousness.

Unless we are enlightened, there are myriad layers of tensions and resisted experiences held deeply in our bodies that our newborn feels, too. Such feelings may begin the contraction and holding in a baby's body that continues throughout life. When we meet our our resistance, emotions can "flower and fade."

It is not uncommon for the body to have its most pleasant memories of being cradled and supported be those times of being held by a grandparent, or some other person, rather than the parent. This is not surprising. Many Children are brought up in isolated nuclear families where we, as parents, often have little or no training in child rearing, and where we may feel anxious or insecure about our ability to look after our baby proficiently.

An obstetrician friend mentioned recently that he often watches new parents walking out of hospital, their day-old baby in tow, with fewer instructions or manuals on how to care for her than if they were walking out of a store with a new DVD player.

Anxiety around parenting can be somewhat compounded if we are older parents of firstborn babies. Especially in cities, we often live whirlwind lives with high expectations of productivity, career excellence, and efficiency—often mingled with chaos, self-criticism, low sensitivity, or too much speed. We might require immediate excellence and perfection of ourselves and our parenting abilities. Naturally, our babies destroy that image fairly quickly, but with some cost to themselves in terms of picking up on the underlying tension.

Maybe our own parents were or still are like that, and perhaps they themselves held us with mild panic and anxiety when we were babies. The difference between a new parent and one who has raised a family can be the sense of ease and patience with which one attends to the newborn. The traditional image of a grandparent as someone with more time to rest and more experience with interpreting baby signals is used here simply to create an image for our bodies of what is helpful for settling a newborn.

Remembering how it felt to be held with a sense of ease as a baby can help us to reconnect to that ease by simply drawing in a couple of deep breaths and consciously relaxing when we are holding our own babies. Finding that place in the body that relaxed when it felt secure and safe allows our babies to feel safe and secure when being held by us.

If we practice this meditation exercise while expecting our babies, we may connect to a memory of how it feels to hold a baby or to be held with ease and confidence. Experiential awareness has a more powerful effect on subsequent behavior than the effect created by intellectually grasping a concept.

Placing my attention there, I become aware of any resistance, any pulling away. I am simply keeping my attention focused on the experience and noticing how, as I allow the experience to flower, so it changes and gradually begins to fade. I can ask the body part that is holding onto this memory what color it would like to draw into itself to help release every particle of the resistance and holding it is still clutching onto.

Having let go of the resistance now, what is underneath? I notice the freedom and openness that remains when I let go of holding and insecurity. What is this experience? I let go even of this question and simply rest with the experience, letting my body soften into the openness. Once again, I take my time with this, noticing how it feels. I sit in a meditative space of easy awareness and attention, bringing my mind back, over and over, to simply how it feels in my body, bringing my attention back to the breath now, back to my surroundings and the room, when I am ready I open my eyes.

Deep relaxation for birth

" To a mind that is still, the whole universe surrenders. "

— Chuang-tzu, Taoist philosopher, 4th century BCE

Relaxation is a form of birth preparation and an important tool for managing the intensity of labor. Not only does it help our muscles work in harmony with one another but it also reduces fear, which produces adrenaline. Adrenaline inhibits the hormones that help birth progress easily. Deep relaxation creates the trance like state that we go into naturally during labor when we are not afraid. Trance happens in the limbic brain—that subliminal, more primal, ancient part of our brain that works together with our autonomic nervous system. Understanding the physiological reasons why deep relaxation helps labor to unfold creates more of a trust in the process, but the experience of deep relaxation is simply one of pleasure of bliss, both for ourselves and for our babies, who are exposed to these hormones when they pass through the placenta.

Our autonomic nervous system (ANS) sends out endorphins, the hormones of well-being, and oxytocin, which starts and maintains labor. The ANS controls the homeostasis in our bodies including: heart rate, digestion, respiration rate, salivation, perspiration,

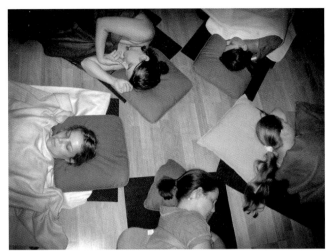

Group relaxation creates a sacred space of peacefulness and serenity.

diameter of the pupils, micturition (the discharge of urine), and erection. These maintenance activities are primarily performed without our conscious control or sensation. Whereas most of the ANS's actions are involuntary, some of its functions work in partnership with the conscious mind, such as breathing. The ANS is governed by unconscious processes, and our unconscious is deeply literal. That is why it responds so well to symbolic language or speaks to us in the language of dreams. HypnoBirthing® (www.hypnobirthing.com) practitioners, who teach a form of deep relaxation as birth preparation, recommend that women refer to their contractions as "surges" during labor. If we use the term "contraction" during labor, our unconscious sends messages to the ANS and the uterus to contract, so that both the cervical muscles and the fundal muscles at the top of the uterus will obligingly contract. This means that instead of the fundal muscles working in harmony with the cervical muscles, pulling them open while the cervical muscles relax and let go, they are working against one another, both contracting and closing down, thus creating rigidity, tension, and pain.

The word "surge" reminds me of waves. Labor surges are like waves, too. They come and go in a rhythmic flow, and we have the opportunity to either ride them or be over-whelmed and tumbled by them. The devotees of a Hindu sage in the 1970s produced a poster with his figure clad in guru robes, surfing the waves. His quote accompanying the image was, "You can't stop the waves, but you can learn to surf." Just so for labor. Staying focused, centered and supported through relaxing, being loved, and feeling safe in labor is like surfing the wave as the surge washes through us. Resisting, fighting, feeling unsup-

121

ported, and afraid of the surge is akin to tumbling underneath the wave, water rushing in through nose and ears, not knowing which way is up or when we'll get our next breath, and finally being dumped in an exhausted, trembling heap on the beach before the next one slams into us. Recognizing this, we can take each surge as it comes, and if we get slam-dunked, our partners can help us to recenter and release the tension that built up through feeling overwhelmed, so that we can ride subsequent surges with equanimity and grace.

Many of the terms we use during pregnancy, birth, and in the early months of our child's life can be invasive and unsupportive on an emotional level. Labeling causes problems to arise simply by our unconscious expectations attached to certain words. Using the word "pain" to describe surges is an example of unhelpful labeling. Maybe your labor will be painful, maybe you will perceive it as excruciatingly painful, but give yourself the chance, at least, to see how you experience it for yourself, before attaching negative preconceptions to it.

Pain is our body's way of telling us that something harmful is happening to us that we need to change—fast. The surges of labor are strong and intense, but they do not feel wrong or harmful when we feel centered and safe ourselves, and when we trust our bodies. The experience becomes one of "pain" when we fight the feeling and try to escape from it, believing that it is somehow wrong and may harm us. Our strong collective expectation of labor pain in our society's consciousness comes in part from thousands of years of imprint-ing that labor is a dangerous business that kills women.

When we were malnourished, with pelvises deformed from rickets; when we had eight or more babies, which increased the chance of post-partum hemorrhage; when we had no access to surgery in an emergency, then labor could be a risky business. Our bones hold fast to these memories, and we are often deeply fearful about birthing babies. However, medi-cal advances and social change haven't decreased our fear of birth. These days, in a First World country, the chance of a mother dying in labor is around twenty per one hundred thousand women. Crossing the street could be more dangerous than that.

Global mortality statistics of four hundred deaths per one hundred thousand women reflect how it used to be before we had medical interventions and good nutrition. There is definitely more reason to fear birth where care and socioeconomic conditions are less than adequate. With proper antenatal care, home birth in the First World is statistically as safe as low-risk hospital birth. As we lose our inherent knowledge of how to birth and how to trust our bodies' ability to birth by allowing doctors to perform Caesareans and inductions with-out medical indications, so our fear of birth and the "pain" of birth increases.

Doctors and midwives who understand this will encourage us to trust our bodies during labor, will encourage our birthing partners to hold us and to help us to soften and surrender into the process. They will provide privacy, quiet, and gentle encouragement and help us feel good about ourselves, our babies, and how we're laboring. Doctors are knowledgeable about birth, but as mothers we often feel inexperienced at it and are supported by partners who don't know what to expect, either. So we need their encouragement and trust, so that we may trust ourselves.

Guided relaxation for pregnancy and to use during birth

> I believe that to have world peace we must first have inner peace. Those who are naturally serene, at peace with themselves, will be open towards others. I think this is where the very foundation of universal peace lies.

— *His Holiness, the 14th Dalai Lama*

Make yourself comfortable.

Gently allow your eyes to close.

Take in a few deep breaths, breathing in calm, breathing out a smile. Feel the smile radiate throughout your whole body.

Very gently bring your attention to the top of your head and begin to feel the sensations in your body. Open your awareness to include the sensations. Notice how, as you place your focus fully on the sensations, your mind begins to quieten down in order for your body to feel with more sensitivity.

Slowly allow a warm sensation of relaxation to seep into your skull.

Feel the tiny muscles around your eyes relaxing, eyes bathed and soothed by this accepting, non-judgmental form of attention.

Imagine the relaxation as a fluid that seeps downwards now through the cheeks and into the jaw. Notice how the many layers of tension held in the jaw begin to soften and release. Feel the relief of allowing the jaw to relax.

The flow of relaxation moves over the back of the scalp and into the neck. Notice any areas in the throat and the neck that might have held unsaid truths or uncompromising attitudes.

>

Breathe deeply into the throat and neck and release any tension held there, dropping the attention lower now, into your shoulders.

Allow awareness to arise as to the amount of responsibility we hold in our shoulders. Softly cradling our shoulders in deep acceptance and awareness, we allow some of that burden of responsibility to be released.

Take a deep breath in and, as you breathe out, feel this burden dropping from your shoulders. Let the shoulders cave in around the trunk of the body as they release their holding. Soft now, as if they were without bony structures, simply notice them softening softening and letting go.

Breathe down the arms—your prana, or life force, is tingling all the way down into the tips of the fingers, bringing an unconditional acceptance into your arms. Allow the cells in your arms and hands to receive this loving attention you are placing on them.

Breathe spaciousness into the chest. Simply allowing sensations of relaxation to flow into the chest, notice how this acceptance and awareness creates a sense of freedom and space within the chest cavity. The breath takes care of us, with or without our awareness, it brings life force into our body. Breathe deeply and easily.

Once more take in a deep breath and, as you breathe out, allow your relaxation to double.

Breathe now into the belly, softening and opening this space that we so often keep protected and armored against the world. Let the softness flow into the belly now, dissolving any rigidity or tension—whole belly releasing, breathing calm and peacefulness into the belly, and feeling this calm flow over the uterus, surrounding and protecting your baby in a blanket of peace. Sense your baby responding to this calm and imagine sending it a color that represents tranquillity and serenity. Let this color flow through and around your baby now, and sense it stretching luxuriously into the peace that pervades your womb and relaxes your uterine muscles.

Feel the ease flowing now, all the way down your spine and back muscles, the whole body sinking gently into the chair, couch, or bed you are resting on, becoming heavier. Feel how, as you relax, so the distinction between yourself and the bed or couch dissolves and softens slightly. Then imagine the stillness descending into your pelvis, which holds and protects your womb. Let go of any tension in this area, allowing it to flow all the way down into the earth where it is transmuted through being released.

Then let the sense of peacefulness flow through your buttocks now and into your thighs. Each area of the body letting go with your gentle attention, knees releasing all tension, calves relaxing and softening, and feeling the life-force energy tingling all the way down into the feet and the toes now.

Breathe in deeply one more time, letting go on the out breath and coming into the present moment, fully relaxed and at ease. Simply resting in this moment, breathing in, breathing out.

Spend a little time resting quietly in the peaceful atmosphere you have created for yourself. Then bring your attention back to the room and, when you are ready, you can gently open your eyes, feeling relaxed and serene, yet energized from the rest you have given yourself.

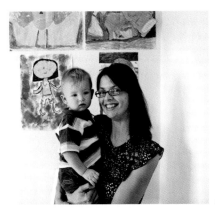

Anakin and Jolene

Jolene's birth story

I feel women should prepare themselves for birth. It's like if I was writing an exam—I would have to be prepared to be able to succeed. I don't mean studying—you have to prepare yourself mentally and physically and emotionally.

I had to just get over my fear of birth. Sometime in life, you're going have to face experiences and to say, I wonder what it could have been like? I had to go the natural way. I didn't have money for epidurals or Caesareans; I was forced into natural birth. I was brought up to believe that birth is the most frightful experience. Just before you die, the baby comes out. A woman is a tough cookie and can take any pain. The most frightening experience I had with Anakin was the moment my waters broke before labor started. The HypnoBirthing preparation, the affirmations every day, all the mind >

training left me, and my body went into shock. It was such an adrenaline rush for about an hour. Then I settled down and when Sue Lees, my midwife, checked me, I was four centimeters (1.57 inches) dilated and I was so relaxed by then that I didn't let it worry me. I wasn't having contractions, just the most beautiful surges. Olivia, my sister-in-law (who is a birth attendant), gave me a remedy to get the surges going. We took a walk around the block, and the surges were really strong. People were so amazed and looking up to us; there was a great respect for us doing a home birth. We came home and Olivia made toast. With every surge I breathed very, very slowly—that did it for me. The surges never went over a minute and a half. Marcus [my husband] came home and Ingrid, my friend, came and they set up the birth pool.

The more intense the surges became, the higher my endorphin levels went. And the happier I became. I was realizing that I was actually doing this, and I was proud of myself. Sue would listen to the baby's heart beat, and she would say, "This baby is loving these surges." She was listening to the baby's heartbeat during a surge, and I was laughing because it felt like someone was tickling me on a high-energy frequency.

I was waiting for the pain, but the pain didn't come. I didn't think I was capable of doing it the way the women did on those HypnoBirthing DVDs—when I watched them, I kept thinking "Good grief, this woman's not even going Uuh!'

When he was coming down the birth path, I made some deep sounds. It was good to make those noises. I never thought I could actually enjoy labor. In the connecting to the unborn child session, Anakin (the baby) said I must enjoy the labor! Whenever each surge was over—you know how when you get drunk, your eyes are all hazy?— well it felt like "drunk eyes" look. Also like when people fall in love. Like when Marcus and I kissed the first time—that high. Not sexual at all, just high. I kept thinking, "Where's the pain?"

In the unborn child session, we spoke about religion. I'm very in touch with God. When I was pregnant, I went back and found out more about the curse that was put on Eve in the Bible—about God punishing women. Well, it's got absolutely nothing to do with having a painful birth, it's all about how difficult life is after the birth, because you give up your whole life for the child willingly. I look at my mother, what she had to go through with three of us …I think that's what God meant. Nowhere in the Bible do they talk of painful births. The only reference to difficult births is to do with breech birth.

I even spoke to my mom and dad about it. If God created me to get so high on my endorphin levels and to be able to cope with labor, why would He make me have a painful birth? Birth is a miracle and why should a miracle be painful? I think the path you walk with your child for the rest of your life is tough.

I think some women are so alone in pregnancy and at birth. They go to their gynaecologistcologist, and he's the only person they see. Women need to know what a doula is. The day that I gave birth, the only male there was Marcus—that day he knew what I wanted, knew how much I'd prepared, and I didn't feel needy of him. He was there, holding my hand and smiling at me when I was having surges, and he was respecting my space.

But with the other women there it was awesome—Sue and Olivia and Ingrid. For my friend Ingrid it was the most amazing experience, as she had two epidurals for her labors. The moment Anakin was born, Olivia was bawling. I looked up as I was holding him on my chest, and Ingrid was also crying—she had an expression of being blown away. She's the kind of woman who needs to be in a hospital for birth, and it was the most amazing thing for her to see Anakin being born naturally.

Olivia was amazing—just the fact that she was so there for me; she didn't leave my side for hardly a second, except to go and pee. Every time I got a surge, she would know by looking at my face; she spoke softly, reassured me, and praised me every time. She gave me more confidence. I would lean over the couch, and she would swing-sway my hips, massage me, ask me if there was anything else I wanted her to do. The surges felt like Braxton-Hicks surges the whole time. Touch for me was very important—just the presence of Olivia and Marcus being there. When I was in the water, Olivia was massaging my back for me. It gave me a better chance. I didn't have to think or worry about anything, I only had to give birth.

Funnily enough, the moment you get hooked on that centeredness and know how to stay there, then it's the easiest thing to do, you can sit back and relax. I wanted the labor to be a normal part of life: the washing machine was on, the TV was playing, everyone laughing and chatting. The laughter lightened it so much. I'm so glad I did the HypnoBirthing, not just for the birth, but for now. Right now as I'm sitting here it's impacting on my life. It changes you.

Visualization

I am awed by the effectiveness of simply visualizing our cervixes opening during labor. We can visualize a flower blooming, butter melting away, or simply a circle getting bigger. Focusing our awareness on our cervixes in a soft attentive way, gives them permission to let go of any rigidity, tension, and holding. Cervixes are remarkably suggestible and open to influence. They really do what they are told, but they are primarily listening to our unconscious messages. To have the most effective conversations with our cervixes, it helps to be deeply immersed in that liminal place that is labor's natural home.

Simply be there with your body, your tender cervix, your baby, your partner, the straggling potted geranium outside the window, and hold them all with a spacious open heart. That is the place where your liminal awareness develops, and that is the place where your cervix can become attentive and respond to your suggestions.

If you imagine the feeling that links you to someone when you are in love, imagine it like a thread of energy—there is a similar thread that links our heart and womb areas; perhaps it has to do with our sexual energy and our affectivity or relationship energy. Link your heart and your cervix in labor. Link them also to your baby and your partner, create a web of love that is all inclusive and spacious, and then watch your cervix respond.

Birth dance

66 Life is movement.
The more life there is, the more flexibility there is.
The more fluid you are, the more you are alive. 99

— *Arnaud Desjardins, French film maker and spiritual teacher* [77]

Dance classes that encourage focused awareness and feeling the music in a physical way can help us move into the trance-like place of birth with ease and grace. A beautiful way to come into a space of harmonic resonance in labor is through dance, as dance can help to awaken life-force energy in the body.

To access this vitality, dancing in labor can be a powerful way to move into that liminal, limbic space of trance while helping us to stay fully connected with our bodies. Dancing in the months prior to labor teaches us how our body feels and how to become

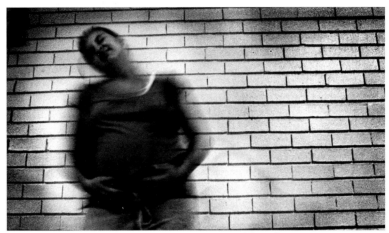

Dancing with our babies encourages prenatal bonding.

more aware of it. We can use it to create a safe space of support and nurturing from our partners both before and during labor.

Dance, when it is employed in a conscious way, reduces the awareness of outside interference and draws us into our senses and our primal and intuitive knowings. This is the place where we discern how to birth with ease and with grace. Dance helps our bodies to soften, to be flexible and open to the process of birth. The warmth and tingling of surrendering can be felt through simply releasing into the feel of music and our body's rhythmic response to it. Each woman can use dance in the way that feels most comfortable to her.

Dance is a fine way to remember how to play—an art that is all but forgotten in too many people's lives. Unlike children, when we first begin to dance as adults, we often produce an initial fear response at simply allowing our bodies to feel the music and move to it. Social conditioning and ideas about what the other people in the room might think of our movements can be inhibiting. So programs like Biodanza start with music that is fiery or has military rhythm to help us expend the adrenaline produced by our fears. Once we've tired ourselves out somewhat, and started to laugh and have fun with the movements, then it is easier to let our bodies soften and become more flexible in response to the music. Dance classes that have been designed for pregnant women and their partners can create an opportunity to receive and give support from and to our birth partners. During labor, dance can help our bodies to open, our minds to fall into trance, and our emotions to feel love and pleasure. Women who surrender into their labors have this dreamy, unfocused look in their eyes, which seem glazed and washed through by the power of birth. Birth eyes remind me of lovers' eyes after kissing, nuzzling, and falling into each other.

Dance during labor can create an intimate bubble of privacy in the middle of a hospital. It can take the form of gentle swaying on one's own or with a partner to deeply surrender into a primal and private space. Dance may create a sensual awareness of our own bodies, and this helps us to soften and open up to release our babies gracefully.

At its most extreme we can dance as wild animal women, who are totally surrendered to the power of birth. Most women shrink from the idea of extreme expression in the labor ward, disturbing the medical staff and possibly their mothers-in-law. But it does raise the question of whether this is purely social conditioning and reminds me of stories we are told of Victorian women who would probably have shrunk from fully engaging in the act of love-making. It also makes me wonder why a woman letting go in labor by expressing her birthing power should be more horrifying than the shrieks of pain issuing from the throats of women resisting their labors?

We can choose to fall into this soft and open space quietly, yielding to the power surging through us, or to respond like Amazons, riding the crest of each surge with force and vigor. These are all appropriate and primitive actions that our bodies instinctively know how to make. In the most non-threatening way, dance can provide an atmosphere of intimacy that is sorely lacking in hospital wards.

Ten or twenty years ago, hospital staff would have been aghast at the idea of using warm water for pain relief or of bringing music or candles or aromatherapy oils into a labor ward; ten or twenty years before that, husbands at the birth or dimmed lights were anathema to delivery-room staff. Stirrups for the legs, ether cones for the breath, and episiotomies for the perineum lent the proper atmosphere to the birth room. So why not begin to introduce medical staff to dance and deep relaxation as positive approaches to having joyful and satisfying births, when we know that all the wonderful hormones produced by any joy we feel cross the placental barrier? This is one way we can ensure that our babies will be carrying a beautiful imprint of their first experience of this world.

Dance as prenatal preparation creates flexibility, an open pelvis, and more trust in our bodies. Dance also helps us love our bodies more. As our bodies respond to music and begin to soften, we can feel their beauty seep into us, even through the midst of our usual judgmental and critical approach to them.

Being touched in a way that creates a merging and an exploration of the boundaries between partners through the medium of dance helps us create an intimate bubble of support during labor. Delicate awareness can lead to a sense of feeling merged with our partners in ways that we may not generally explore outside of a sexual context. Trusting that we can be held and supported in this way, in a studio filled with music and other prenatal dancers, gives us the confidence to later allow ourselves to be supported in a loving way by our partners during labor.

Originally, belly dance was created as an exercise for women to teach their pelvises to be flexible and open for labor, and pregnancy was an important time for practicing belly dancing. It only became an art form when men decided it was sensual and designed for their pleasure. The sensuality of belly dancing was the attitude that helped laboring women surrender into the experience of birthing their babies.

Jolene tells us about her ecstatic birth experience on page 125. She was very in touch with her body and says, "I did the belly dancers' teacher training a few years before Anakin's birth, and I love dancing. With belly dancing you have to understand how your body works. If you were to see me before I started belly dancing and before I conceived him, my body looked very different. When you're dancing, *dit voel so goed!* It's so empowering to shimmy."

Toning and singing

" If you want the truth, I'll tell you the truth,
Listen to the secret sound, the real sound, which is inside you...
The music from the strings no one touches. "

— *Kabir, Indian mystic, poet, and saint 1398-1448*

Toning creates an experience of sensing a vibrational openness in our bodies. It has an effect on our physical, mental, and emotional well-being by synchronizing brainwaves and creating a harmonic resonance in the body. This tends to deepen our connection to the energetic patterns around us and within us. By focusing on the sounds resonating deep within our bellies, we move easily into a meditative state of being.

Toning is a system of simply allowing one's voice out while breathing easily and fully. Relaxing the jaw and the belly produces resonant sounds that help us loosen up and that are tremendously empowering. Sounding a single vowel during an extended out breath creates toning. There is no melody and the only rhythm is the rhythm of the breath. When toning in a group setting—often referred to as chanting—one person will begin with a particular vowel sound. This may be a simple vowel, such as "Aaaaaah" or a combination of three sounds, such as "Aaaaa-uuuuu-mmmm"—or Aum. The rest of the group then join in on their out-breaths, simply starting and beginning each sound as their own out breath begins and ends. In this way, a circular rhythm is created with all the individual sounds blending into one long chant.

Toning as a group can be satisfying and release inhibitions around our voices. In the same way as football chanting creates group cohesion so that the sound seems to emanate from one organism, so toning as a group gives one confidence in one's own sound because it seems to blend in with and belong to the whole. It is also possible to tone on one's own.

Toning doesn't require training or an ability to sing. I was brought up to believe that my singing voice was genetically impaired and that people would laugh at me if I tried, but even I allow myself to tone. Creating sound by vocalizing a note heals us on physical, psychological, and spiritual levels. Once it begins to resonate through the body, our whole being begins to hum with vitality.

One of the best places to learn how to tone is in the bath. The water helps the sound to reverberate back to you so that it sounds richer, your head can rest back against the edge of the bath, relaxing the jaw, and the rest of the body usually unwinds easily in the bath, too. It is a good place to practice without worrying what other people might think of you.

Open the mouth by dropping the jaw and allowing it to recede slightly so that you look like the imbecile you might feel like shortly. The tongue can rest on the lower teeth. Focus the attention on the belly, either at the solar plexus or preferably lower down, near the hara—four centimeters (1.6 inches) below the navel or even lower down at the perineum. Breathe in deeply and release the breath a few times, and then, on a long out-breath, allow a deep sound to emerge from the belly.

Initially it might sound as if it's coming from the throat, but as you continue, if you focus on dropping the sound into the body, you should gradually become aware of feeling the sound beginning to emerge from the abdomen. Relaxing and opening the chest like a barrel helps the sound to drop into the diaphragm. As you relax the belly and focus there, you will feel as though the sound is being produced by the belly itself, and it will begin to resonate there. When this happens the quality of the sound changes and becomes richer.

We are in no way trying to make beautiful sounds; we are only trying to find our own sound. Some people are natural sopranos, but we all have the ability to tone deeply, and it is the deeper frog-like or mooing sounds that help open up the lower chakras, ground us, and help the cervix to open in labor.

Birth companions can be a great support in using toning during labor, by making toning sounds that harmonize with our sounds and that help us feel less self-conscious. We labor best if we are centered in a deeply limbic space inside ourselves. It is not easy to follow intellectual instructions from there, but we can follow guidance or being shown how. So birth companions can help us to open up energetically in labor by toning together with us rather than by telling us to tone.

Chanting has been used in the East for thousands of years to encourage meditative states and enhanced states of consciousness by repeating phrases while toning. San tribes in the Kalahari sing and chant to encourage tribe members to move into trance states. I have only recently begun to work with sound and pregnant women, but I am very impressed with its potential to support women in labor. Dr. Michel Odent, French natural birth consultant, has long emphasized the advantages for women of singing during pregnancy to bring their bodies into harmony and balance.

I am awed by how obviously babies recognize sounds from their prenatal experience. They turn to gaze at fathers when they hear their familiar voices. Babies love songs that have been sung to them in the womb, so if they recognize songs they often focus intently and visibly relax.

Rhian gave birth to Anela at home. Her labor was hard, and Anela was upset after birth. She yelled intermittently for half an hour until Stuart began to sing to her. She paused in her crying and looked deeply into Stuart's eyes. Rhian joined the singing, and for the next half an hour while Rhian was being sutured for a perineal tear they sang this ancient melody. Anela was entranced, gazing back and forth from Rhian to Stuart, clearly recognizing a tune that had been sung to her in utero. Her breathing settled, her little body relaxed, and she fell into the singing and into her body in a trusting way that indicated that she felt safe here.

I attended a meditation retreat recently where the two monastics leading the retreat had beautiful voices. One of them sang lullabies to us during a deep relaxation session, and the atmosphere in the room softened into a deliciously nourishing space. I felt safe and cherished as the singing wafted over me. So now I've taken up singing lessons. Me, the one with the defective voice! I want to learn how to pass that feeling on to mothers, so they may pass it on to their babies.

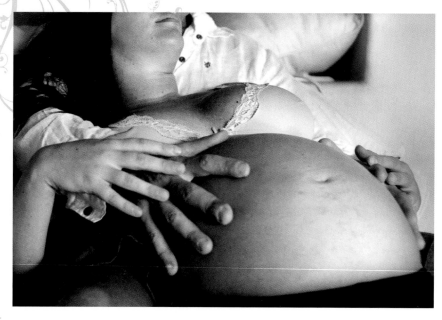

Touch and massage

We have an essential need to be touched with affection. Affective touch releases tension and gives us permission to trust our surroundings. The Touch Research Institute at the University of Miami collated studies on the benefits of touch and massage. They found that, "Massage therapy during the first fifteen minutes of every hour of labor decreased anxiety and pain and the need for pain medication. In addition, they found that the massaged mothers had shorter labor, shorter hospital stay, and less depressed mood,"[78] and that "Labor pain is reduced by massage therapy."[79]

Another study showed "decreased anxiety and stress hormones (norepinephrine) during pregnancy and fewer obstetric and postnatal complications, including lower prematurity rates, following pregnancy massage."[80]

Touch and massage can help us to move into the limbic, interior world of labor. If we are held and soothed in labor, we are helped to feel supported to trust what is happening in our bodies. There is a very strong mind-body principle at work during labor, and the more we trust and let go, the more easily our labor progresses. During pregnancy we can receive touch from our partners and from massage therapists.

A womb recreation session can help us surrender and release tension in our bodies that has been held there since childhood. As with any kind of deepening work, the quality of attention of the supporters and the creation of a safe space to work within are essential for any relaxation to occur. Therefore, the space must be quiet and undisturbed. Telephones should be disconnected and switched off. Soft background music, soft lights, and soothing aromas that are safe to use with pregnant mothers help to create an atmosphere of peacefulness. The focus of our attention should be calm and clear. It is always beneficial to practice some form of deep breathing and relaxation or meditation before beginning.

The purpose of this exercise is simply to create a place of deeply supported relaxation. Taking turns in groups of three to five, have one woman lie on a couple of soft blankets or a comforter on the floor. The others sit around her, each placing their hands gently yet firmly on one of her limbs or on her head. Spend four to five minutes, or perhaps the length of a relaxing piece of music, to allow the woman to gently "unwind." Each of her movements is supported and held by the hands of those about her. At the end of each process, spend a couple of minutes breathing quietly, simply holding and supporting her body, before she exchanges places with another member of the group. This exercise helps us loosen up safely. As our bodies learn to open and relax, so they remember what that feels like. This reawakened memory can be accessed during labor to facilitate softening and opening.

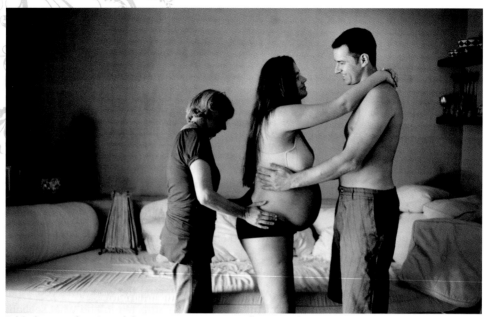

A birth attendant's task is to encourage a good connection between birthing partners.

improved when women are supported and feel safe due to the presence of doulas during labor. Women tend to have fewer medical interventions, fewer Caesarean sections, fewer birth complications, and their babies are healthier, more content, and breast-feed more easily. These might seem like inflated claims, since doulas simply contain the space in which women labor, but the vastly improved birth outcomes make more sense when we remind ourselves of the impact that our hormones have on birth. We know that fear causes adrenaline production and high levels of adrenaline coursing through our laboring bodies can result in physiological spinoffs, such as fetal distress or stalled dilation. Epidurals, while minimizing fear, can numb us emotionally as well as physically and can detract from birth's transformational potential. Statistically, they have been shown to impact negatively on bonding and breast-feeding.

A doula does not replace our birth partner; she acts in a supportive role to both parents, and her role is to encourage the birth partner to recognize how integral their involvement can be in creating a satisfying birth experience. Part of a doula's role is to assist the partner in staying more involved during labor, rather than pulling away during times of stress. Because doulas are familiar with the process of birth, they can honestly reassure both parents about the normality of the experience during times when it might seem overly intense.

The power of birth generally has a long-term impact on our emotional and spiritual well-being. Whether it creates a positive or a negative impression depends on our circumstances, our level of trust, and our ability to remain open to the experience.

A doula's work is to simply pay attention every moment to exactly what we need, identifying when to soothe, reassure, listen, or build confidence, and when to encourage us to connect with our partner and our babies. Each moment of full support and attention we receive assures us that it is okay to yield to birth's power. Feeling that we are held with deep attention in the labor room gives us permission to trust that we are being cared for and watched over, and that we are safe in what is often unknown territory and uncharted depths. Sometimes we need a pair of hands to sway our hips, sometimes the encouragement to feel our partner's love, sometimes a lullaby or some firm direction to be brought back from a place of fear or panic. Whether we need laughter or a place to wail or groan reveals itself moment by moment and is infinitely variable in every labor.

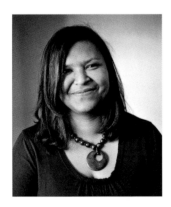

Lana

Interview with Lana, mother of Luca and a birth attendant

I was a home birth. Being a woman of color in those days meant you were born at home. Gynecologists were reserved for affluent women.

My mother wasn't serious when she described my birth. She said my dad was excitable but not helpful. He kept trying to mop her brow with a cold cloth and smothering her. He was so excitable that the midwife had to ask, "Do you mind if I have a chance >

here please?" to move him out of the way a bit when I was being born.

I didn't fall pregnant easily. I was working in a clinic weighing babies and listening to other mothers' birth stories. They were all about how something awful had happened to them, and none of them trusted their bodies. I think all the women with good births just stayed home and didn't come to the clinic; you hardly saw them.

I wanted a home birth, an intimate experience. Whatever I wanted, Glynnis, the midwife, made me feel it was completely okay and doable. I was a week overdue and was so excited when I went into labor. We didn't worry about time during the labor; I was able to move around. She didn't dictate how I should hold Luca after the birth or how I should feed her, either; she just handed her over to me. The environment was so under my control.

The moment she was out I felt, "Oh my gosh. I have done something exceptional. I am so clever!"

I started attending births a year later. The first one was for a single mom under state care because she wasn't working. She was induced. I couldn't believe how awful it was. The women were all left alone; there was no compassion. It was a real abuse of women in vulnerable situations. Support people were not allowed in for any of the other women in labor. Nothing I did seemed to console her, anyway. After that I trained for one year in how to support women more effectively.

The best birth I attended was a home birth soon after I had completed my training. I was still working at the clinic then, so I arrived after 5 p.m. to the smell of oils and candles. I came just at the right time, as she started with strong surges. The baby was finally born at three the next morning.

Every touch I offered she found helpful. She just wanted to hold her husband's hand. I was watching the midwives and how they work. I don't know what was so special about the birth—I think it was her sheer determination, her courage, and her calmness. She was exceptionally focused. After the baby came, the midwives had to eventually push me out the door to go home and get some sleep before work the next day. Afterward, she said that the touch was what helped her most.

Another birth I remember as being extraordinary was very vocal. It was also a home birth. Afterward, the neighbors came by to congratulate the mother because they felt they had been so involved through the birthing noises. I think using sound during labor is underestimated.

None of the fathers have ever felt I was taking over their role as support person. We all work as a team, and they are grateful for someone there to reassure them and to support them in supporting their partners. I've met very few men who feel able to be sole support.

I think mothers who birth naturally feel more positive about themselves. So I am there to help them achieve that. With hospital births, a doula is often the only person in the room to keep a calm environment, to make it safe and warm and nurturing. I supported one woman through labor simply by holding a facecloth against her forehead, and she told me four days later that she could still feel my presence in the room. She knew I was there, and that's what made her feel calm. The babies can feel it, too. All they need for the birth is a sense of presence, of everybody being right there and focused on the birth. That's what makes it calm and happy for them.

Peaceful birth visualization

Bring your attention to your body, make yourself comfortable, and when you are ready, gently close your eyes.

Feel the muscles in and around your eyes relaxing—all the tiny lines around your eyes releasing and letting go. Eyes bathed in a soothing fluid of relaxation. Take in a couple of deep breaths, breathing in calm, breathing out a smile. Allow the smile to extend beyond your lips, and feel it releasing tension from your eyes, breathing in calm, breathing out peace… slowly in and out, awareness settling into the breath, breath deepening, flowing smoothly and gracefully through the body.

Imagine a balm of soothing relaxation flowing in through the crown of your head and softly soaking through your body, releasing any tension as it does so. Feel this warm soothing sensation moving from behind your eyes into your jaw—jaw receding slightly, tongue resting gently against your upper teeth, relaxation seeping into neck and shoulders, shoulders caving in around the form of your body, all the muscles in and around this area becoming soft and loose. Deeply relaxed now and moving even deeper into a place of stillness and tranquillity—body, mind, and emotions coming into perfect harmony and balance. Any thoughts that arise drifting by without your mind attaching to any of them. Mind's attention placed on the quiet, calm sensations in your body.

>

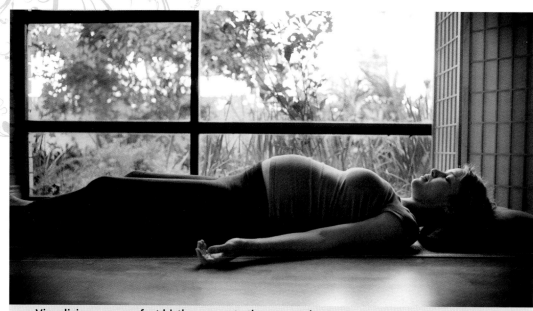

Visualizing your perfect birth can create the unconscious conditions that allow it to unfold.

Relaxation moving farther down into your body now, chest releasing and becoming more spacious as the tingling sensation of relaxation opens the whole area. Notice how the borders and edges of your body soften and dissolve slightly as you allow your body to relax; your body feels heavy and when you place your awareness on the sensations of your body touching the couch or bed you feel the connection firmly. Feel the couch or bed holding and supporting your body.

Let the relaxation flow farther down your body into your belly, belly softening and releasing any tension. Mothers feel the relaxation flowing around your baby in your womb, visualize your baby enjoying the peacefulness of this moment and, enjoying the spaciousness, the muscles of your uterus relax. Feel the pelvic bones that support your belly and uterus releasing any tension, so that they hold your womb in a soft and supportive embrace.

Relaxation moving farther down now into your thighs, knees, calves, and feet. Relaxation tingling all the way down into your toes—legs, which carry you forward in life, simply releasing and letting go, no need for their muscles to do any work at all at this moment. No need for you to go anywhere, to be anyone, to do anything. Simply being in this present moment, with relaxed and calm awareness.

Imagine you are in a special place in nature now—your favorite space. Visualize the colors, the sounds, the atmosphere. Is it warm or cool? Can you feel the breeze on your skin? What details do you notice about this place that makes it special for you? What is the ambience like? How does it make you feel to be in this place? Name how you are feeling quietly to yourself. Find a couple of adjectives to describe the feeling of being in this special place today. Where in your body do you relate to the feeling of your favorite space? Feel the sensations of peace, joy, trust—the ambience you have named—in your body part.

Allow yourself to move now to a place in the future when you and your baby are moving through the extraordinary experience of birthing with gentleness, tranquility, and calmness. See yourself as you will be during your birthing in a place of true empowerment—so centered in the middle of your labor. Breathing calmly with each surge, remaining centered, focused, and present, and sinking deeply back into a place of deepest serenity and peace in the spaces between the surges. Surges ebbing back and forth, flowing with them—focused and centered. Then deeply, deeply relaxed in between. Feel the sensuousness of your connection with your body, your baby, and your birth companion. Notice the connection between your baby and yourself as you move even more deeply into relaxation. Feel the connection between all three of you—yourself, so calm and centered, your baby in the perfect position for birth, maneuvring her way downward, your birth companion so caring—holding you in this safe, supportive place. Feel your connection to the earth—her feminine compassionate energy keeping you present.

How would you would like to experience your birth? See yourself enjoying the birth that will be completely perfect for you. What is it that you and your baby will choose in order to have this perfect birth? What will you be feeling? Experiencing? What will the atmosphere of the birthing room be like? Name the qualities of energy that you choose to feel at your birthing time quietly to yourself. Name the sensations you would like to experience in your body. Notice how easily and smoothly your baby will slip down the birth canal and out into your arms.

See yourself now in the moments after your baby will be born. See your birth companion with you as you hold your baby close to your body, skin touching skin, connecting deeply to your baby and yourself. All three of you bonding and deeply connected. Feel the joy of finally meeting your baby—this baby that you both connected to while in the womb. Aware of being able to feel the smooth creamy vernix on your >

baby's skin, touching it delicately, amazed at the sense of presence and calm awareness emanating from your baby. Surrounded by the warm atmosphere of birth, the
smells, the closeness, the quiet, peaceful dimness of the birthing room. Notice the
timeless, undisturbed atmosphere. Your baby lets you know when she is ready to have
her connection to your placenta cut. Notice how wonderful it feels to respect your
baby's knowings in this way.

Drink in the atmosphere of this birth that will take place for you exactly as you have
imagined it, because you have created an intention for it to unfold in such a perfect
and wonderful way.

Spend a moment or two more simply staying present with the awe and wonder of
this moment of birth. Then when you are ready bring your attention back into this room,
knowing that you have imprinted your perfect birth firmly in your unconscious mind.

Feeling so peaceful yet alert, so calm and centered, so at peace with allowing the
rest of the pregnancy to unfold in its own time, at the perfect pace, so that when your
baby is ready, you will all three experience this perfect birth. When you are ready, you
can open your eyes.

Integration therapy empowers birth

> One does not become enlightened by imagining figures of light,
> but by making the darkness conscious.

— *C. G. Jung, Swiss psychiatrist, founder of analytical psychology* [83]

Integration therapy is a simple tool for becoming clearer, more focused, and more centered
in life. It embraces many different levels of awareness, including sensations in the physical
body, emotional feelings, mental focus, and spiritual depth. When the awareness extends
beyond a personal sense of self, our relationship to the outer world is also seen as an interdependent part of our experience.

The sessions may be used for understanding why we are experiencing difficult situations, in order to release the energy that creates those circumstances. They are also used
for connecting with our unborn children or for releasing fears that we hold around birthing

and parenting. Integration therapy brings a more holistic approach to birth and can make the experience of birth more profound by encouraging an awareness of the myriad levels of reality that are influencing the birth and are impacting upon it. The safety and security offered by medical advances in obstetrics over the past years have given women the courage to be able to focus beyond the physiology of birth and to be able to embrace the power of the birth process more fully.

Closing down to the emotional impact of a less-than-perfect birth creates emotional jarring that can remain held in the body in a timeless sort of way, alongside all our other life events and traumas. Emotions have a sticky quality, and unless we actually work through them, we suppress them deep inside our cells. This eventually influences our perception of the world and creates negative patterns of behavior. Birth is a *big* moment, and its immensity can be perceived by mother and child as either terrifying or empowering. Its impact on our life is similarly huge.

Yet if we bring even a modicum of love and welcome to our babies they are still far more soft, expansive, open, and responsive to life experiences than we are as adults. We can see this in their tiny bodies, which are so free of tension. Babies are unaware of themselves as separate beings, and from their perspective they, their mother, and their surroundings are one being. They are still living from their center, and they express this in bodies that are flexible and free of resistance.

When they encounter difficult situations such as a sore tummy, they begin the process of building up resistance, tense their bodies and arch backward against the uncomfortable experience. As life goes by, so the resistance in our bodies and psyches builds up, until our responses to the world around us are largely conditioned by these resistances. The layers of our personality and character arise from our conditioned behavior and often from our instinctive urge to avoid the same painful events we have encountered previously. These incidents may arise from this lifetime or possibly from our genetic inheritance or even from previous lifetimes.

A session, usually of two to three hours, involves us using deep relaxation to access the imaginative stories held deep within our bodies. The facilitator's role is to ensure that we feel safe and trust the process. During an integration session we are assisted to work with the unconscious, irrational parts of ourselves, which are rich with stories. This is the place where we weave our life experiences into a tapestry upon which we play out each new experience.

Every previous encounter informs and directs our attitudes and approaches to our unfolding life. As Shakespeare so rightly told us, "All the world's a stage / And all the men and women merely players." We script our lives based on our loves and losses, our expectations, hopes, and dreams. Connecting to the scriptwriter is like having direct access to humanity's consciousness. In releasing personal, intimate specifics at this level of reality, we see that our own holdings and resistances are the holdings and resistances of humanity and that we have within us the potential to be a saint, rapist, politician, wise woman, or the guy next door.

There are no promises or expectations with the sessions. We never we know at the start of the session where we will be led. However we do know that because the sessions are guided by our own intuitive deep knowing, we will only look at the experiences that we are ready to release. As a result, the sessions feel safe. It is the extent of our willingness to surrender into the process that determines the amount of benefit we receive from the session. Sessions, therefore, require that we are willing to take responsibility for our lives and our part in the creation of the circumstances in which we are living; on the level at which we work, everything is so interdependent that our input into the world in which we live totally changes and molds the form of that world.

The energetic changes that occur from sessions impact our external environment. In her session, Joyce recognized a mean and abusive man as holding a similar relationship with her as her neighbor in her everyday life. She hadn't spoken to him for very many years as a result of an argument they'd had. Arriving home after the session, she was preparing lunch, prior to mentioning the contents of her session to anyone, when this neighbor phoned. Please could he come over later, he asked. He felt it was ridiculous that their feud should have lasted so long, and besides he had a book that he wanted to lend her.

We may feel the emotions that arise from any of life's potential experiences in a session. Like actors who live and breathe their roles and become their characters for the time they are on stage, we have the opportunity to experience aspects of life that we may previously have denied ourselves.

A woman who, during a session, experiences herself as a manipulative martyr controlling her family through her passive anger and her "poor me" attitude is able to release the potential she has for this type of misuse of her feminine energy. In doing so, she is able to more fully claim her feminine power and use it more creatively and enjoyably.

Or the timid, shy girl-woman may experience herself during a session as a vampire seductress with blood-red lips and huntress eyes. She finds she is mistrusted by other women, and she uses her sexual energy to control men and have power over them. In releasing her very real knowing of her potential ability to use her sexual power in this damaging way, she is likely to allow herself to enjoy her body, her sexuality, and her pure femininity without fear of hurting or controlling others.

Janine experienced herself as a servant girl, being used as a sexual object by her "master." In her "story" she falls pregnant and is sent to jail by the mistress of the house, who is jealous of her. The dominant feelings in the story are of being used by people she admires because they have so much more than her, and she also experiences a strong sense of powerlessness. In releasing these feelings, which are held in her pubic area, she feels a soft, warm flood of love in her heart. Her heart welcomes it "like it's been waiting for it a long time." There is a sense of a warm red color "filling and filling" her whole body.

The beauty of the work arises from its symbolic content. In everyday life, stories are just stories, but from a deeper level they are significant and archetypal. Symbols illustrate the content of our thoughts and emotions, but they can also transcend them and our ability to analyze them. They work within the deepest recesses of our brains, molding and transforming us.

Regressing to birth can sometimes be part of the process of integration therapy. I once worked with two men on the same day, both of whom reexperienced their births. The first had been born at twenty-eight weeks and lived in an incubator for the following six weeks, completely separated from an extremely ill mother. The second was unwanted. It seemed that the greater trauma was experienced by the unwanted baby. The child in the incubator was absolutely certain of the love his mother felt for him, from her bed in the Intensive Care Unit. His experience was, in fact, one of compassion for her, since she felt so bereft of her connection to him. The unwanted child felt isolated and abandoned, even though his birth was normal and he was kept with his mother in the hospital.

The adage, "as within, so without" is very true in the context of this work, and as we become less complicated and more centered, so the complexity and emotional drama of our lives decreases, and we find ourselves living in a more contented, light- and love-filled world.

Rachel was studying integration therapy with me in Amsterdam. Her two children had stayed behind in Israel with her husband, Arik. It was the first time she had ever left them and Yoni, her youngest, aged six, was struggling with the separation. Rachel felt guilty and uncomfortable at being so far from them.

Two weeks after Rachel had left home, Yoni developed a raging temperature, with no easily diagnosable symptoms. For four days he was feverish, and Rachel, who was understandably worried and distressed, was ready to fly back home. So we decided to do a session clearing her relationship with Yoni first. In the session, Yoni was furious with her, so we worked with that, and Rachel released that energy between them. Twenty minutes after we had completed the session, Arik phoned to report that Yoni had woken forty-five minutes ago—just at the time we were releasing the energy—he was completely better and, in the way only a young child can accomplish such a miraculous recovery, was running around the house behaving as if he'd never been ill at all.

Integration therapy is employed during pregnancy to clear individual fears and negative expectations for the birth process itself. Our minds have a powerful effect on the process of birth. Fears about labor, birth, and child rearing dramatically affect the birth itself. These fears may be caused, for example, by generational and cultural beliefs, television, something our obstetrician told us, advice from friends, or possibly from the consciously forgotten, deeply buried memories of our own births. They may be held deeper still, in the collective memories of our culture's psyche and in the memories of our mothers and grandmothers, which are passed down to us genetically. These fears can be so deeply ingrained on an unconscious level that we are hardly aware that they are there.

Unrecognized themes are inevitably passed onto our children in a long stream of descendancy, which the Dutch refer to as *"De Rode Draad,"* or "The Red Thread." I am drawn to this description. It evokes images of women's cycles, a menstrual history that passes from generation to generation, a legacy we live out through our children and grandchildren. It is as strong and as unconscious as our most primal instincts. These memories are not vague ephemeral wisps floating in the ether somewhere; they are held in the cells of our bodies— in our bones, our blood, our hearts, and livers. With acknowledgment and work, we can release those aspects of the Red Thread that no longer serve us or our children. In doing so, we let go of patterns of behavior that have been entrenched over the generations through fear, patriarchy, and a disbelief in our own natural power.

During sessions, we are guided by our own intuitive wisdom to recognize the themes we are carrying in this lifetime. The sessions can be undertaken by pregnant women, postpartum women, and partners of birthing women. Since we are in charge, it can be an empowering process. The facilitator's role is to keep us safe and to guide us to our own intuitive understanding of where we need to go. As in birthing, where laboring women seldom require more than help and support to let their own bodies tell them what to do, so in integration therapy work, the facilitator allows our "Higher Self" to show us aspects of our lives we need to clear most.

Often we may choose a "past life" to express the theme we most need to clear. I'm never absolutely certain whether the "past lives" are actual lives we experienced or whether they are simply convenient stories to illustrate unconscious fearful attitudes that have locked us into negative patterns of behavior. No matter. The changes that occur in our lives after we let go of themes we have been clutching onto for years in the mistaken belief that these protect us convinces me that it is irrelevant to our lives now whether they originate in past lives or are illustrations of traumas experienced in this one.

Beneath the layers of resistance from our many different life encounters, we are, in our core, unchanging, deeply wise, and unconditionally loving. Our true nature is the same as our neighbor's true nature. Literally, from this level of consciousness and experience, we are all one. At the point of intersection between our true nature and our personality or self-conscious aspect, is a place of deep stillness, where we can access wisdom and intuitive guidance. From this elevated perspective, we are easily able to uncover those resistances that cause our negative patterns of behavior. In releasing them, we lead our lives from a more centered, less reactive perspective.

An enlightened person is one who has released all their resistances to life—who has no reactive patterns to their experiences but responds fully and openly to each and every situation. If we could stay fully open to new experiences and release those we have suppressed as a result of resisting uncomfortable feelings that arise in us from them, they would simply flow right through us, without sending reverberations and reactions back into the world. The process of integration therapy is to work with these layers, one at a time. The purpose is not to become so enlightened that we can levitate, develop paranormal powers, or be worshipped and admired by our peers. It is simply to help us negotiate our way through life with a bit more grace and equanimity. As a result, the people with whom we interact are no longer bombarded by the "ripples and earthquakes" of our reactions to their negative behavior, which are reflected back at them.

We can develop our ability to birth and rear children in an instinctual, loving, and confident way. By connecting with our children, born and unborn, we learn to trust their higher wisdom to help guide us in their birthing and rearing. Once we have acknowledged the intuitive wisdom we all hold within our bodies and psyches we touch a core consciousness, which we recognize as being our inherent birthright. In working with this wisdom, we come to understand its intrinsic quality and see that it is not a learned process of acquiring knowledge but rather an honoring of a collective wisdom that is greater than ourselves, a wisdom that, being ageless, belongs to our children as well. Recognizing that, we are able to trust enough to release authoritarian, controlling attitudes for child rearing. Instead, our children's upbringing becomes a dance of listening, engagement, negotiation, and guidance.

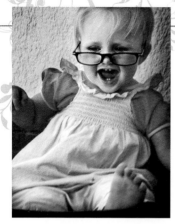

Jeanette's daughter Kano.

Jeanette's difficult birth

Jeanette did a lot of work with her unborn child and with clearing past issues while she was pregnant. She had a difficult birth and her baby needed incubation for a time afterward.

She remembers the sense of timelessness around the birth as being so vast.

The jump from pregnancy to having a baby is so huge that you move into a state of limbo. It's the biggest jump you experience in your whole life. There is no rational process taking you from one to the other; the only single thing that connects it is the birth.

The unborn-child work was awe-inspiring, breathtaking—to see her, touch her, hold her, smell her before birth made me feel so ready.

I found the surges during the birth so amazing. Then it went so wrong. There was meconium in the amniotic fluid, and eventually she went into fetal distress. There was so much fear at the hospital with the gynaecologist and everybody running around. Fear for the baby and for me.

I had a sense of not being contained, a sense of being dropped. However the fear was around me but not inside me; the unborn-child work took away any fear of giving birth or of pain—the fear was depleted and it was the most natural thing I could do.

When she was born she was blue. There was something wrong with her—I couldn't hold her or nurse her. I was so weak for the next two days; I was in and out of consciousness. The pediatrician thought she would spend months in ICU, but after two days she was fine. He thought it was a miracle. The amazing part is to trust that.

It took me a long time to recover from the birth experience, and now I can say we are fine. But the thing is we were fine all along. Despite all the drama and the problems, it's been so natural. It wasn't easy, but it was special and almost indefinable despite all the early troubles.

It was almost like giving birth to a part of you, an extension of you but in another form—like we know deep down that we are all the same in essence. Well, that feeling of being so connected to another being was clarified for me through the sense of giving birth to such a special creature.

Being a single mom and not having my mom around, I used to have the fear of transposing my mother's fears and insecurities through me onto my baby. But the unborn-child work gave me the knowing that I would be able to hold her and nurture her own development and her own personality and being without allowing my own and my mother's stuff to cling to her. Our connection being untainted by past trauma, I was able to enjoy and experience and feel her while carrying her and during the birth experience. The sessions gave me a clean slate. I still have a slight fear of tainting her with my past, and sometimes I catch myself on a day-to-day level. But the moment I interact with her there's none of that; it's completely pure because the fear isn't there then.

She's a profound little creature, with these angelic smiles that make you just crumble. She's my teacher. She creates the opportunity for me to learn an acceptance of everything that is true, of what is; it's not grey and darker grey, it's black and white. She's got a clear-cut idea of what is right and what is wrong, and she shows it to me with such a passion.

Her name, Kano, means "knowing." I always thought I would have to meet her first before I could name her. One day the name came up, and now I understand why— it was kind of preparing me for what I was getting. And her second name is Perth, which means "initiation." I knew this was her name, and I knew the meaning; I just didn't understand the implication!

It's that smile. She presses and presses and presses me, and then she smiles and it all just melts. When I say press I don't mean she's difficult or demanding or temperamental; I just mean there's an intuitive knowing that when you get close to her you are exposed to essence. And it exposes everything in you that is not essence, and when you feel "I don't know anymore. I can't do this anymore; it's too much," she just smiles a smile of unconditional love, like she's wrapping you in a blanket and it's all okay.

Conversations with our unborn children

We do not cause the imagination or deserve it, yet it is intrinsically part of us and sustains us every day.

— *John Tarrant, Zen Buddhist psychotherapist* [84]

One of the most uplifting experiences of pregnancy is to work with forming a relationship with our children when they are still in the womb. Unborn babies are so connected to their soul's knowings that they hold a wisdom that far surpasses our narrow, limited version of reality. Shortly into any session working with unborn children, they reveal themselves to be filled with unconditional love and to have a deep acceptance of us and our inability to understand life from their much clearer perspective.

Pregnancy is a time of spiritual connection. If we choose to do so, we can generally experience our spiritual reality more profoundly and easily than at other times of our lives— perhaps because our babies have an expanded sense of awareness, and we are physiologically, psychologically, and psychically interdependent. As Rhian said in her session with her unborn child, "It's almost like I can see the connection between my heart and womb where the baby is; there's this strong red force connecting us. She's a naughty, cheeky elf with a grin and then a laugh like music."

Rhian's sense was that her baby was such a happy, giggly being that she wanted lots of laughter to make the birth easier. The session made her feel "calm but strong at the same time." Her husband Stuart, who attended the session with her, described his connection to their baby thus: "It seems like a glowing white ribbon from my heart. Like a longing. I can't find words for it. It's just love; bursting-at-the-seams kind of stuff." I emailed Rhian to check if she was okay with me quoting from her session, and in her reply she added; "P.s. funnily enough, she is like a little elf with a grin that wins you over, and everybody comments on what a happy baby she is, so my unborn session rung true!"

Parents' inner wisdom guides them to feel this connection to their babies. Even those parents who don't trust in their ability to connect intuitively to their child in the womb seem to easily establish this relationship once they relax and allow the process to unfold. As they soften, listen, and feel the quality of his essence, the baby then tells them what he needs to say. He may even encourage them to look at relationship issues. This can create a healing in the family dynamic and can resolve themes prior to the baby's birth, rather than as life lessons later.

As a facilitator, it is remarkable to watch a baby guide her parents to look at their negative patterns of behavior. It would not be considered helpful for me to tell a mother during pregnancy that her nagging, for example, or her anxiety, perhaps, is having a negative effect on her relationships in general; yet, she will easily accept such advice coming through her own mouth from things she "imagines" her unborn child is telling her. She will not only accept such advice but also will happily work on an energetic level to release these patterns and move beyond them to a more loving sense of self. It can be enormously helpful for the birth experience to make a connection with your child before your expected date of delivery.

Sebastian was so sure of himself in his communications with Sarah prior to his birth. (See the interview with Jono and Sarah on page 186.) He had a real sense of being centered and calm and sturdy. He had no particular requirements for the birth itself and told Sarah she could do whatever she liked for it (a home birth with a birth pool, a midwife, birth attendant and her husband Jono in attendance) because he would be absolutely fine, anyway. Today, Sebastian is six weeks old, and Sarah has this to say about him, "The information he gave me was absolutely accurate. He really did say how it was for him. He's such a solid, strong little guy. He has no feeding problems and is putting on weight much faster than Ollie did. The sense I get most from him is one of calmness, a feeling of 'I'm here and I'm okay with this earth experience.' My connecting with him before birth was also wonderful for Jono; he found it much easier to get a sense of Sebastian's presence once I described the experience to him."

Often the birth partners also choose to attend this prebirth session. They relax deeply during the session, especially if they have prepared previously during antenatal preparation with guided visualization for relaxation, and they are either included in the session, experience it as an observer, or sometimes they go on their own journey with the baby. Birth partners almost always find that the experience helps them to know how to help the mother focus on the type of birth their baby suggested would be helpful for everyone during the labor. The sessions just prior to birth are rich and filled with meaning for the parents. When our babies show themselves to be wise in such a profound and non-judgmental way, it can change our relationships with them forever. We may later forget this when they are being horrid and demanding toddlers, but developing a multidimensional view of who these beings are does have a deep-seated impact on our future relationships with them. Conversations with our unborn babies help us as parents to connect to a deeper level of reality, and sometimes to a sense of the oneness underlying our concept of reality.

Karina's baby expressed this to her as a huge beam of light that surrounded them during the session and which she asked Karina to remain aware of during the labor and birth. She requested that her father Tom, the midwife, and Karina all stay connected with one another and with her through the birthing by focusing on this light.

The extraordinary advantage given to women who connect in this way with their babies prior to birth is that the births are then baby-directed. We know from scientific research that when birth is left to follow its own natural course, it is the baby who physiologically sends out hormones that trigger the start of labor. Since it is, after all, his birth, not our own, it seems sensible that he has more say as to the manner in which he will be birthed and received into life.

Nathan, as an unborn child, told Dudu, his mother, that he needed lots of time to birth. She connected with him during the early phase of labor, and then she labored in a manner that dawdled along, albeit with Nathan's head so well descended that it was almost pressing on her perineum, and she finally birthed him three days later, when he eventually decided to slither out into the world. If we hadn't listened to Nathan's request for more time, Dudu would have slipped into the hospital system's management protocols with augmentation of labor and intervening in its normal process. Studies by perinatal psychiatrists on how birth experiences relate to our everyday perception of the world indicate that this might have created a difference to Nathan's outlook on life.

During the sessions, babies will present themselves as a quality of energy experienced by the parents as sensations, feelings, and emotional attributes; often they have colors surrounding them. They may even take on symbolic form, like a star or a radiating ball of light, rather than always taking the form of an image of a baby. They are sometimes gentle, sometimes strong. They can be funny, joyful, calm, loving, or steady. They are always wise. Even a mentally challenged child will be profoundly wise at this level of connection, and could explain some of their purpose for choosing their handicap.

Babies' birth choices are usually simple; they may ask their mother to trust in the birth, to surrender her fear or her need to control the process, or ask that they be held with patience and attention in the weeks after the birth as they settle into their life. Yet because mothers are so deeply in tune with their own unconscious processes during the session, it becomes a simple matter for them to release the fears, the need to control, or the impatience on a subliminal level, so that these patterns of behavior are unlikely to impact on the birth or newborn period.

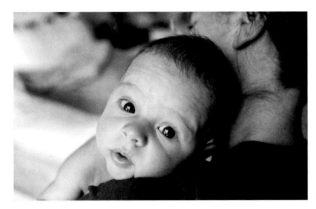

Gabriella and James.

Gabriella and James –
Talking to Michael, their unborn child

Gabriella and James helped their baby, Michael, to heal a physical hole in his heart, through their unborn child session with him. The hole in his heart had been identified at a fetal assessment center a few weeks prior to their session. During the session, we focused on the images arising from the anomaly in his heart area to see whether there were any unhealed emotions that could have been a contributing factor.

Gabriella – imagining her favorite place in nature at the start of the session:
It's like a clearing, and there's a huge waterfall in front with lots of really green plants around a clear pool. Mist from the waterfall is spraying on me. I'm standing on the side, about to enter the pool. My feet are in the water. I can hear the birds and the crickety insects. It feels warm, but I'm not hot. All the leaves are wet—a dark, shiny, green color. It smells like it just rained. It smells like birth and rain mixed together. It smells very clean. It's a nice place. I've been here before. It's very calm and tranquil, and it feels safe. It also feels like it's hugging me. It's very nice, very peaceful. The water is still, even though the waterfall is dropping into the pool. The noise of the waterfall is not too loud. There are little bits of sun coming through the trees above—not too sunny, there is lots of shade as well.

James's favorite place: *I'm at a beach. On very white sand. I'm sitting up against quite a large, cool rock. It is warm, not hot. I can hear waves in the background, they're not loud. There is the sound of seagulls and the movement of a gentle breeze. The colors are just before sunset—deep pinks and reds. It feels very peaceful* >

and serene and comfortable. I am on the sand. The smell is salty, lightly salty with a bit of seaweed smell in the distance, and a smell of shells and the sand.

Gabriella – connecting to her Higher Self or the symbolic form of her core essence: *It's just a round ball, like what the sun would look like, with light coming out. Quite large and energetic. All the colors are light, like whites and yellows. The center is white, and then it's yellow. It's like glowing; radiating and not moving around—moving within itself. It's good. It's very strong, very powerful. It's got a very clean and pure energy. It touches mainly on my chest, which feels nice, feels warm. It feels like as if I take a deep breath. It creates spaciousness and a softening, which spreads down my shoulders.*

James – connecting to his Higher Self: *It looks like a heart shape, and it's a similar color to the white light, except it's more sparkling. It seems like an energy on its own, very strong and powerful and very pure. It sort of sparkles. I would say its energy is that of power, self-assuredness, and just like a brilliance. It touches my head, my face. It feels like when you are in a bath: you put your head under and warm water is completely surrounding you—warm, gentle, and all-encompassing.*

Gabriella – being given a tool by her Higher Self that can help her in her life at this moment. *It says peace, symbolized by a bird, a dove. It is white and in my heart. It feels nice, very peaceful.*

James – being given a tool by his Higher Self that can help him in his life: *It's like a flute of sparkling, almost shimmering powder that I can bring into my mind, and whichever path I walk down I can sprinkle it, and it can add beauty and change and light and awareness. It feels like it is in my brain and in the thoughts that I think and in the roads that I walk down; it creates beauty. The things around me start becoming the same color. They sparkle, become clearer, more beautiful, and I feel happiness and peace.*

Gabriella – a message from her Higher Self: *It says I must relax, and I mustn't worry.*
James's message: *Enjoy. I must enjoy every day.*

Gabriella – on connecting with Michael, as her unborn child and allowing his consciousness to take form: *It looks like a little baby. All gold. It's just floating in front of my Higher Self. It's still little—about three weeks old. It's naked, glowing, and it's also turning around slowly. It's bouncing a lot now; it's a happy baby. It's bouncing on its bottom; it looks soft. My Higher Self is protecting it. Emotionally it's very good, very strong and powerful, very happy. It's a nice baby.*

James's unborn child: *It's also a naked baby. About twenty weeks or so, curled up, floating above my Higher Self in the same white light. Turning around slowly, looking very happy and peaceful. It seems to be of the same form as my Higher Self —peaceful and loving. This feeling comes from the baby. It spreads out in all directions, like a vibration. The baby is Love.*

Gabriella – on looking at her baby's heart: *I think the hole is still there, but it's not so bad. I can see it glowing, it's still dark in the middle.*

James's baby's heart: *It's a little, tiny, black area, very small, on the right-hand side of the heart. It looks as though the heart is a very deep pink color. The hole is a tiny area almost like a bit of black in the veins on the skin. When the black stuff is sorted out, the hole will close.*

Gabriella – on looking at the moment in time when the hole first formed: *It was right at the beginning. There are round cells, and some of them are popping —it looks like bubbles. It's real. There's anger. I'm unhappy, inside and outside, everywhere—I can't identify where exactly. It feels like a big weight, squashing me everywhere. It's very heavy.*

Both Gabriella and James identify the moment as having occurred during an argument they had when their unborn baby was tiny. They then ask the part of their body that is holding the memory of the hurt and anger experienced during their argument what color it needs in order to be released. Once a suppressed emotion has been identified and the sensations of the emotion have been experienced, it is more ready to be released from its entrapment in the body. Since each color holds a different frequency of energy, and our bodies know exactly the frequency of energy that will facilitate each particular emotion's release, we can ask our body which color it would choose in order to let go of a negative experience.

Gabriella draws blue into her heart area, which is experiencing these feelings, and this helps to clear the heaviness out. *It feels a bit better.*

James – on looking at the moment in time when the hole first formed: *It was also like what Gabriella said; it was very early on. We were arguing about something, were very unhappy about something that was happening in our lives. I'm feeling discomfort. I feel that my muscles are all very tight. I feel like I have a bit of a headache. I feel anger. I feel fear. I feel hurt and disappointment. I think I feel them in my heart.*

James's heart chooses blue to clear the feelings held there. *It feels better, cleaner. The black stuff that came out when I washed my heart is the same stuff that is on the baby's heart.*

>

Gabriella: *It's smaller.*

James: *It looks like it's gone.*

Gabriella uses yellow to clear hers completely: *It's broken into little dots. It's gone.* [She looks at her baby's heart.] *Its heart looks nice. The baby has lifted its head and is looking. It looks happy—its eyes are smiling.*

James: *The hole is almost closed now, and there's a white clear membrane, a tissue on the inside of the hole; it's going to grow together. It's the beginning of the closure of the hole, and every day it's going to just get stronger.*

Gabriella – on asking her baby what it needs from her for the birth: *It wants me to be calm. I feel dizzy.* [She grounds the energy and feels better.]

James – for the birth: *I need to be a calming influence.*

Gabriella asks her baby what gift it would like in order to come into harmony and balance with her: *Love and peace. It's like a blanket. It's yellow. It's melting into the baby. He looks very happy.* [They hadn't been told the baby's sex. Gabriella correctly refers to Michael as "he" during the session.]

James's gift to his baby: *Love and tenderness, like a soft knitted blanket. It looks like a scarf—it's wrapped around the baby. The baby relaxes more, becomes calmer.*

Baby Michael gives Gabriella a gift to come into harmony and balance with her: *It's giving me love. It really loves me. It looks like a lot of ribbons—pink, blue, green, purple, and yellow, all mixed up and glowing. It feels good. It tickles, makes me feel very nice. I feel much better than before.*

James's gift from their baby: *The baby reached out and put its hand around my finger and left like a clear Perspex around my index finger, and it started to go different colors—pink, orange, and green. This feeling of connection just spread through my whole body.*

Gabriella: *It says it's happy and that it loves me and that I mustn't worry.*

James: *It says just to enjoy this time, because if I enjoy these days then Gabriella will enjoy them, and the baby will, too.*

Gabriella drew her Higher Self into her chest: *It feels like peppermint!*

James drew his Higher Self in through the top of his head: *It feels like the rushing of air, and now I feel complete again. The baby said about the birth that we're all in this together. We're all going to go through the birth together.*

Six weeks later, at their follow-up fetal assessment, the hole in Michael's heart had closed, exactly as he had promised it would if they cleared the energy that had created it. James and Gabriella have a very close relationship. They continued working on any differences in their outlooks after their baby's birth. And each time they found a new way to keep their communication between one another clear and open, they would notice the difference in how much more smiley and relaxed Michael had become.

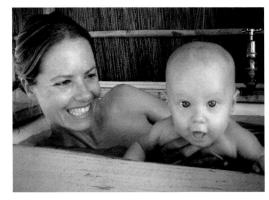

Mel and Ethan.

Mel and Wolf connecting with their unborn child

Mel and Wolf attended their unborn-child session together. Transcribed below are their imaginings as they were guided through the session. A session always adapts itself and changes form according to what unfolds as it progresses.

Mel – on imagining the connection to her Higher Self or inner wisdom after first spending a little time relaxing and deepening her awareness: *It looks like crystal quartz in area under my heart. It feels like if I've made a good decision then it shines; lights up the area. Fear suppresses the shine. I need to give it space, my chest helps to lift it, gives it space, whereas doubt or fear closes it in.* [She allows it to radiate out.] *It's warm and light. It's lifted—a trusting feeling, and open as well.*

[She asks the crystal quartz to lead her to the consciousness of her unborn child.] *I'm feeling a fear, like stage fright. My heart energy is pulsating; it radiates out. It feels trapped if it can't radiate.* [We work with this trapped feeling, which soon dissipates.]

>

On feeling the connection through her Higher Self to her unborn child: *The energy in my belly where my baby is feels like it just likes being here, it's peaceful. Soft, very soft* [her voice becomes very soft] *like a little lamb. It's just soft—it's like very pure. It's lying there, happy to check the world around it. Not afraid at all.*

Gift from the child to come into harmony and balance with Mel: *Surrender. It's showing me how it's a soft little lamb, yet it's not afraid of the world that it's in. It's happy to lie in the field. It's just happy. Wagging its tail very fast—in bliss, as it feeds.* [She draws this feeling into her heart and starts to cry.] *It feels like excitement; like the best thing in the world.*

Mel's gift to her unborn child: *A sense of excitement. It just knows this feeling. So much happened since I've fallen pregnant* [she was hospitalized with a deep vein thrombosis for five days when she was five months pregnant]. *Worries, concerns. I didn't have the sense of excitement at the beginning.*

How can she support the baby during birth? *It's again just trust, and there's that same feeling—be in the space of softness and surrender. I feel it in my belly.*

Where does she feel mistrust? *In my hips.* [She washes this energy out with the energy of trusting.]

How can Wolf (her partner) help during the birth? *I just saw a glimpse of his facial expression after we swam with dolphins in Mozambique—his happiness to have experienced what we did together. He can bring that happiness to the birth.*

What does her baby need after his birth? *It's related to my upper chest* [the quartz crystal feeling of light radiating out] *like it just wants to share in this quartz crystal— light-filled, open, radiating.*

Deep vein thrombosis? *I'm just visualizing it as dark, stagnant blood.* [She surrounds it with the energy of the quartz crystal, which symbolizes her inner wisdom, her body's knowing.] *I'm partly wanting to blast it with light. Something in me says its okay as it is. Something else I'm getting—an acceptance of what's not perfect, the dark. It's okay, and there's so much that's life.*

Message from her unborn child as the lamb: *Just I'm getting that it likes to bask in the sunlight.*

Wolf's feedback of his process after the session, which he was participating in silently: *Such lucid imagery. Like a curtain opening in the darkness. Lucid, three-dimensional images of dolphins in the water. So lucid when I was in the experience; then, when I became conscious of myself, I would lose it.*

There was another plane beyond that: Like in a space movie, traveling through space through a hole—an organic shape, flattened and tapered. An electric blue space cloud—very lucid. I was aware that these are the bands in which dolphins travel through space and time. Blue-electric-smoke-liquid.

Wolf's connection to his unborn child: *It's a bright spark; multi-multi-colored, incandescent, a rainbow is primitive—it was the whole universal color spectrum. A dolphin-deer-lamb-dragon being—gentle, though. Then I moved into fears and uncertainties for a while, a messy, untidy space. My body is under so much tension—layers and layers, on a day-to-day level. There was like a torrent of energy trying to get through my body. Towards the end of the session I relaxed; through the breath I let layers go quickly. Mel's talking about the radiance of the child filled me with happiness. Light, incandescence.*

Mel's thrombosis: *I had a parallel experience, of wanting to blast my fears and uncertainties with light, and then seeing the "ism" of the space I'm in and accepting it just as it is as well. The torrent of energy wanting to come through my body was like the baby wanting to be born through the constriction of fears around birth, which can hamper the birth of a child.*

The lamb basking in the light: *I saw the eye only of the deer-dragon-wolf-dolphin face. It had the most beautiful doe like eye, with long eyelashes. Like a deep soul, looking into its eye.*

When Mel was crying: *There was a parallel again with my own life; how I conduct it. I was in a simple space of just observing. I noticed that I need to look and to appreciate my emotions more. There's a level of un-emotionalness. It was such a beautiful feeling; such love for Mel and the baby.*

Mel and Wolf's story – After the birth of Ethan

Mel: *At times, I felt as though my birth was a medical case study. Everybody wanted to induce me or do a Caesarean because of the deep vein thrombosis (DVT) I developed during the fifth month of my pregnancy. Finally I met Dr. Hume, who was very knowledgeable about DVT and advised me that the best way for me to give birth was naturally, and that a doula would increase my chances of achieving that. He supported my wish to give birth in the hospital in Hermanus with Tilla Miller, a GP who attends many births there. The birth itself was wonderful—almost a home birth. I think the* >

best part of the labor was the first part. It was just myself and Wolf, and it taught me to listen to my body—what position felt right and to focus on my breathing, learning to trust ourselves and each other.

Wolf: *It empowered me to call on my gut feelings. Next time we would like to have a home birth.*

Mel: *Induction would have robbed me of my confidence in my ability to give birth. I think the important thing about birth is to stick to at least a little bit of what you want, and you can do this in almost any circumstance. I think we look outside of ourselves so easily for the perfect birth, thinking that candles, music, etc. would create it, but it is all inside of you. Perhaps it doesn't matter so much if you're in theater with bright lights and so on, if you can hold onto the beauty inside of you. We were playing a dolphin sound track at home, and it continued in my head the whole time I was in hospital, too. Leaving hospital so soon after the birth (an hour and a half later) was special, too—to go back home with Robyn as our midwife and settle into our own bed.*

The unborn-child work changed our relationship to the birth, and made it more intimate. Once he was born though, you just see him, and then it's not so important anymore.

Wolf: *It was good in that it set the team up and got everyone onto the same page. It was a releasing experience.*

Mel: *Also it taught me not to have fear. The unborn child as a lamb didn't have any fear. Especially when I was in hospital, that came back to me often—how unafraid he was. So during labor I didn't have any fear, which helped tremendously with dilating so fast.*

Wolf: *It was so mind-blowing how Mel surrendered into the birth. I wanted to tell you about the synchronicity of Ethan's day of birth according to the Mayan calendar and the unborn-child work. The dolphin symbol was so powerful during that work, and Mel wanted dolphin music during the birth, and we both really connected to the dolphins in Mozambique when Mel was pregnant. Ethan's Mayan glyph for his day of birth is Chuen, which denotes innocent spontaneity, and its symbol is a dolphin.*

Ethan was hospitalized for a urinary tract infection at about two months.

Wolf: *The experience definitely deepened the connection between us. He would gaze into my eyes until we found a still-point. My calmness was able to keep him calm. I really got to see how brave and strong this little guy was. All he wanted was to know he was not abandoned.*

Mel: *I don't want to make out that hospitals are negative. The birth experience in hospital was positive, and hospitals are necessary; we are grateful for them. Ethan is incredibly calm. He's such a happy baby. He first smiled during his first week—looking at us with a really engaging smile.*

Wolf: *His attention was always there. He was incredibly aware immediately.*

Mel: *He's got such good manners.*

Unborn child meditation for pregnancy

It is more valuable to connect to your unborn child with a trained facilitator, as each session is adapted to what the child brings. However it is possible to get a taste of the connection through this simple meditation. First read through it yourself, and then ask someone you trust and feel comfortable with to read it aloud to you. Let them take their time and read slowly. They can wait for you to answer them aloud after each question. Ask them to transcribe your answers for you to refer to later.

Unborn child meditation

Make yourself comfortable. Gently allow your eyes to close.

Take in a few deep breaths. Breathing in calm, breathing out a smile. Feel the smile radiate throughout your whole body.

Very gently bring your attention to the top of your head, and begin to feel the sensations in your body. Open your awareness to include the sensations. Notice how as you place your focus fully on the sensations, your mind begins to quieten down in order for your body to feel with more sensitivity.

Slowly allow a warm sensation of relaxation to seep in through the crown of your head.

Feel the tiny muscles around your eyes relaxing. Eyes bathed and soothed by this accepting, non-judgmental form of attention. Eyes feeling held and at peace.

Allow the fluid of relaxation to sink downward now through the cheeks and   >

into the jaw. Notice how the many layers of tension held in the jaw begin to soften and release. Feel the relief of allowing the jaw to relax.

The fluid of relaxation moves over the back of the scalp and into the neck. Notice any areas in the throat and the neck that might have held unsaid truths or uncompromising attitudes.

Breathe deeply into the throat and neck, and release and let go of any tension held there. Dropping the attention lower now into your shoulders.

Allowing awareness to arise as to the amount of responsibility that is held in the shoulders. Softly cradling the shoulders in deep acceptance and awareness, we allow some of that burden of responsibility to be released.

Take a deep breath in and, as you breathe out, feel this burden dropping from your shoulders. Let the shoulders cave in around the trunk of the body as they release their holding. Soft now, as if they were without bony structures, let them relax and soften. Breathe down the arms—the prana, or life force, tingling all the way down into the tips of the fingers, bringing an unconditional acceptance into your arms. Feel how the cells in your arms and hands tingle and thrill to receive this loving attention you are placing on them.

Breathe spaciousness into the chest. Simply allowing sensations of relaxation to flow into the chest, notice how this simple acceptance and awareness creates a sense of freedom and space within the chest cavity. The breath takes care of us, with or without our awareness; it brings life force into our body. Breathe deeply and easily.

Breathe in a feeling of peace. Breathe out calm acceptance. Fully open to this moment exactly as it is. Embrace this moment.

Bring your attention into your womb. Softly, gently, begin to notice the sensations in and around your womb. Become aware of any sense you may have of color in the womb area. Move into this color and feel it surrounding you. Move deeper into the womb noticing any other colors that may arise and that you move through.

Find the color that feels comfortable, special, and supportive to you. You may like to choose one of your favorite colors or simply imagine a comfortable and supportive color. Breathe that color into your womb area, and surround your child with it. Feel a sense of trust developing as you relax into this color. What does trust feel like to you? What can you trust in yourself? Can you trust the love you feel for your baby already? Can you trust the way you relate to a specific person, animal, or place? Ask your body what trust looks and feels like? Does it feel warm, supportive, rich, creamy, soft, or strong? Develop the sensation of trust in your body. Find your own images and sensations to describe this trust to yourself.

Trust that this feeling that you have created and connected to in yourself can show you an image of your core self—that unchanging, uncontaminated, wise, and pure inner being that resides at the center of each and every one of us. Create an image simply by imagining one. Let an image or symbol form in your mind that expresses this inner being for you. It may take the form of an angelic being; it may take symbolic form or a form from nature. Notice the first glimpse of an image as it arises. Don't question it—simply allow it to be by imagining its qualities. Dwell on and slowly develop the details. If you were to describe its qualities what would they be? Allow the qualities to express what you imagine your perfected form would take. If you can't trust that you are able to create an image in your mind, imagine a color that represents your Higher Self, or simply imagine and then feel the sensations that such a being would stir up in your body. Let the energy of this Higher Self radiate toward you and touch your body. What does it feel like?

Ask your Higher Self to show you an image of your perfect birth. Describe what you imagine, either to yourself or aloud. Now reconnect to the color surrounding your unborn baby and ask your Higher Self to show you the consciousness of this child in this special color.

It may take the form of a baby, or it may take on symbolic form, like a star or a radiating ball of light. Take your time, and allow the first fleeting image to gradually develop and become stronger as you pay attention to the small details you imagine belong to the consciousness of your baby. What colors are there surrounding him? If he's a baby, what is he wearing? How old is he? What do his feet look like? His expression? His emotional quality? Is he joyful, sparkly, or quiet? If your baby has taken on symbolic form, what is the quality of energy like? What are the colors? Do they radiate, sparkle, glimmer, swirl, or are they quiet, calm, and gentle? Feel the emotional quality of the form.

Feel the energy of this being touch your body. Recognize the connection. How does that feel in your body part?

Ask your unborn child what he would like to have for the birth, to help him birth in the way that will leave him with the most positive imprint as his first experience? How would he like you to be during labor and birth? How can you work together? Get a sense of how to support him best. Imagine the color that would support him at >

this time and would help maintain your connection until the birth. Send him this color from your heart.

Let the consciousness of your child now reenter your womb, and feel the energy of it within your baby in your belly. Feel your connection to this wise and precious being. When you are ready, bring your attention back to the room, listen to the sounds around and outside. Breathe in and out deeply. When you are ready, open your eyes.

Birth Ceremonies [85]

Entering motherhood is a very important rite of passage, which deserves to be marked and celebrated. Celebration of marriage, death, birthdays, bar mitzvahs, or twenty-first birthdays is commonplace; yet, there are few appropriate rituals with which to commemorate the powerful transition into parenthood.

Rituals pay tribute to each new stage of life, by marking a particular moment in time with significance and meaning. Birthing ceremonies honor the archetypal wisdom within women and create a context for surrendering into the primal journey of birth and motherhood.

The most important element in creating a birth ceremony is that of bringing conscious awareness into the meanings and symbolism offered by each ritual. As in any rite, it is the intention behind the ritual that creates the depth and significance of the act.

Many women find that while baby showers are a wonderful acknowledgment from their friends of their upcoming birth, they wish that they could celebrate it in a more meaningful way. Pregnant women often feel very drawn to ritual—to consciously connect to themselves, their babies, and to a spiritual dimension in life. Rituals bring power and meaning to the passages between different stages in life and create a bridge between inner experiences and the external world. A birth ceremony is a woman-centered celebration that especially focuses upon the strength, beauty, and transformation of the expectant mother.

Birth is a time of transition from the state of girlhood or womanhood to motherhood, and the ceremony can honor what the mother is leaving behind as well as what she is about to embrace. It can represent a symbolic "birthing" of the mother. Fears and doubts can also be remembered and released.

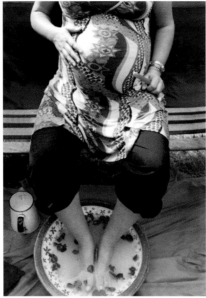

Ernie's birthing ceremony.

Ceremony preparation can be organized by you or by significant people in your life. Since birth ceremonies often replace baby showers, they are traditionally but not exclusively, arranged by other women in the community.

There are many options available for your ceremony, some of which have been listed below. Consider them in the light of the intentions and symbolic significance they convey. Simply holding a short ceremony in a place that feels sacred because care and love has been taken with its preparation can make a deep impression on the participants.

Design your ceremony with the following factors in mind:
Time: Consider when you would like to hold your ceremony. Do you want to hold it on the day or evening of the last full moon before your baby is due to be born? If that is too New Age for you, perhaps you would prefer to choose a time for purely practical reasons. Would you prefer to hold it during the first trimester as a celebration for the pregnancy?
Who is the ceremony honoring? Is it for yourself, both you and your partner, for your baby, and do you want to acknowledge her siblings?
Who would you like to have present? Do you want women only? Friends? Family and relatives? Only significant people? Would you like children to attend? Would you wish to invite the caregivers who will be present at the birth? Will guests have specific roles?

Where would you like to hold the ceremony? Will you have it indoors or outdoors? At home, or out in nature? Choose a place you love and make the space special by decorating it with flowers. If the energy of the space is important to you, you may choose to cleanse the space before the ceremony. Create a warm and safe environment. Will there be a focal point like a fire? A circle can create a powerful holding space reminiscent of a womb.

How would you like people to participate? Would you like participants to read poems, prayers, affirmations, or stories? Would you like to include dancing, singing, meditations, or visualizations? It can create a wonderfully warm atmosphere to have guests participate through painting your belly or through creating gifts for you and your baby during the ceremony.

Would you like to use ideas from traditional ceremonies? For instance African ceremonial rituals might include the creation of a beaded necklace. New Age rituals may include invoking angels or goddesses.

What kind of atmosphere do you wish to create? An intimate space? A holding womb like space? A nurturing space? A space of laughter and celebration? How will you create the atmosphere for the ceremony? Candles, aromatherapy, music, food, flowers?

How much will participants be involved in the ceremony? It can be more meaningful for guests if they also prepare for the ceremony in some way—with wishes for you and your baby or with gifts.

Rituals

Be aware of the meaning of each ritual for you when choosing rituals for your ceremony.

• **Create birthing necklaces or bracelets with birth beads.** The purpose of a birth necklace or bracelet is to remind women either of the links among their friends, who may or may not have birthed before, or of the link among all birthing women over generations. As such, there are two ways you could perform this ritual: Each woman attending the ceremony brings a bead representing each child she has birthed, along with their birth stories, which are told as each bead is threaded onto the necklace. You add your beads, first for previous babies, and then one for the upcoming birth, to the necklace. The necklace is placed ceremoniously around your neck, with blessings. You may choose to wear it continuously until the birth occurs, or to save it to wear during the birth itself, to serve as a calming focus and to remind you of your link with the other women who are emotionally supporting you at this time. If there are women among your circle of friends who are unable to conceive, they can place a bead on the necklace for their yet-to-be-conceived baby. Alternatively, the entire necklace can be threaded with beads representing each woman's aspirations and blessings for you and your baby. A necklace can be created that gets passed from birthing mother to birthing mother. Before your ceremony you choose, find, or create a special bead to symbolize the pregnancy, birth, and life-to-come with your baby. This bead is added to the birth necklace, which is entrusted to you at the birth ceremony to wear or keep until after your birthing; thereafter, you record your birth story in a journal that accompanies the necklace. The necklace and journal are then passed on to the next pregnant woman in the community at her birthing ceremony. The journal is filled with the birth stories of each mother who placed a bead on the necklace, their purpose being to inspire, uplift, and empower the birthing women who follow. The journal and necklace hold deeper meaning and become richer over time as more stories, beads, and experiences are added. Difficult births may be recorded in a way that helps to heal and to recognize the spiritual significance of the experience. As such, the journal becomes a book of wisdom, shared teachings, and connections to the upcoming generations. Even if you are the first mother to create the necklace, it is possible to add your bead to a thoughtfully chosen cord and begin a birth necklace and journal for other mothers following in your footsteps.

- **Create a beaded necklace for the baby with each bead representing a wish or blessing from guests at the ceremony**
- **Create a "web" of sisterhood.** You sit in the center of a circle, and a ball of cord or wool is passed across you repeatedly to link you to the wrist of each woman in the circle, creating a web of connections. The cord is then snipped and a piece of it is tied to each woman's wrist as a reminder, to wear until after you have safely passed through the birth time.
- **Hair brushing, foot washing, or foot massage rituals.** These can serve to make you feel special. Flowers can be woven into a wreath to place around your head to wear during the ceremony.
- **Birth stories offer personal testimonials about birth.** These provide an opportunity for your friends to share their wisdom and experience with you. This may need to be guided to ensure it doesn't end up being a disempowering list of how gruesome birth was for women in situations where the birth was medically managed and choice was taken away from the birthing mother. Blessings and good wishes from each participant are often offered at the ceremony for you and your baby.

- **Have a poetry reading.** What poems would you choose, or will participants bring poems?
- **Build a mother nest.** Each participant can bring something special to add to your "nest" to help create a safe space within which to give birth.
- **Movement and dance can express joy, gratitude, and blessings for you**
- **Gratitude prayers and giving thanks**
- **Mindful meditation**
- **Write a communal letter to the unborn baby**
- **Create a mandala symbolizing community, the circle of life, the thread of wisdom passing from generation to generation**
- **Do belly painting.** Each guest has an opportunity to apply face paints to your belly to decorate it and to create a belly "art piece," which can be photographed afterward to remind you of your connection to each person who added to the painting. Henna painting is usually done in preparation for the ceremony. Choose one or two people to decorate your belly with henna—women who will make beautiful marks so that you feel special and gorgeous. Incorporate music and singing into your ritual. Which music or songs do you wish to include in your ceremony?
- **Gift Giving** may be incorporated into the ceremony, together with blessings from the giver.
- **Food** may be brought to share or may be provided by the host of the party or yourself.

Arrangement and order of the ceremony

Having chosen the rites that you will perform at your ceremony, decide on the sequence of events. Will you have somebody officiating?

A typical ceremony may include:
- Welcoming
- Opening the ceremony, possibly invoking a sacred presence
- Introductions by each person present
- Nurturing you as the mother
- Offering of blessings
- Creating a symbol
- Completion
- Feasting.

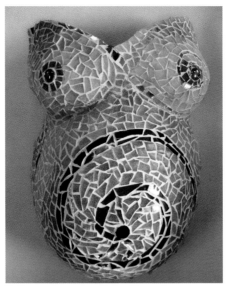

Belly casts are a celebration of our beautiful pregnant bodies.

Belly Casts

Celebrating pregnancy by making a cast of your belly is a wonderful way to prepare for birth and to feel good about your body—the same body that can be tiresome when it's achy and sore and heavy, especially in the last few months of pregnancy. Belly casts are fun to make, and can be interesting and revealing to decorate with symbolism that relates to the pregnancy, the baby, or the birth. And they're beautiful. I have yet to meet a mother who hasn't admired her belly cast as a remarkable sculpture. They are smooth, round, feminine, promising. They lend themselves to appreciation and adornment. They assist women in feeling beautiful about themselves.

Wait until the last two months before your baby is due before you decide to make your cast. You will need someone to help you since you will be moving as little as possible during the process.

You will need:
- Five to six plaster of paris—impregnated bandages, about ten centimeters wide. If they are narrower you might need seven; if they are much wider you could do with four and cut them in half. Don't buy ordinary bandages and plan to dip them in plaster of paris

yourself. The consistency is difficult to get right and they slip off the body, don't hold their shape as easily or get lumps stuck on them

- Cotton wool or cotton batting
- A box of plaster of paris for smoothing over the casts afterward
- Vaseline
- A bucket of warm water
- A pair of scissors
- A tray to lay everything on
- A kikoi, reboza, sarong, or towel for tying beneath your belly.

If it's a warm day, consider making your belly cast outdoors. Plaster of paris washes off easily if you clean up immediately afterwards, but belly casting is a fairly messy business.

Cut the bandages into strips of between twenty and forty centimeters (8 and 16 inches) long. Smother your belly and breasts thickly in Vaseline. The cotton wool needs to be able to stick to the Vaseline, and the plaster of paris then sticks to the cotton wool.

If you're using cotton wool, gently separate it into sheets that are half or a third the thickness of the cotton wool. If you can do this, the cotton wool works better than the cotton batting, and thinner sheets mean that you get a belly cast that is closer to your actual belly contour. If the cotton wool is too thick, you can lose belly button bumps or nipple shapes. Batting, while thinner, has more defined edges, which are more difficult to approximate with each other.

Your helper places a layer of cotton wool over your belly and breasts. Cut or tear the edges to fit closely together. Stick the cotton wool to the Vaseline on your belly as far back as a perpendicular line drawn from your armpits. Be generous with how far back you place the cotton wool if you want a full belly. Too far back of course, and you might have to wait in your cast until after the birth, to shrink enough to be able to get out of it! The cotton wool can be placed just above the level of the pubic hair underneath your belly, and can follow the shape of a bra line or bikini line on your breasts. Again be fairly generous. You can always pare it down afterward before it gets too dry. Check that you have placed the cotton wool evenly on both sides of your body, comparing the edges by feel.

Settle yourself in a position that you can maintain for about fifteen minutes to half an hour. Some women stand, some sit on the edge of a birth ball, some adopt an upright reclining posture against a deck chair. If you lie flat on your back, the size of your belly cast will be significantly reduced. Your helper needs to be able to reach underneath your belly to fix the lower layers of bandages in place. Some women choose to lift their arms and rest them behind their heads to lift the breasts away from the belly somewhat; others choose to have a more natural posture for their casts.

Your helper holds a strip of plaster of paris at either end, dips it in the warm water, and places it on your belly. The strips don't have to follow any particular direction, although you will need to have a few layers of strips that follow the edges of the cast to make a stronger frame. He or she should keep placing layer upon layer on your belly until the whole belly and the breasts have been covered with at least three to four strips in each area. By now the cast will be beginning to dry and hold its shape. Your helper can gently knock on the cast to hear the hollow sound of areas that are still weak and thin.

Once complete they can gently lift the cast off you and place it in an area to dry for about half an hour, while you shower to get the Vaseline, bits of cotton wool, and drips of plaster of paris off your body.

Trim the edges so that they are even on either side and the height of the breast edges is the same. At some stage you can add a layer of plaster of paris powder, mixed with a little water into a cream like consistency, if you wish. This will smooth off the bandage texture.

Let your belly cast dry for a couple of days before continuing to work on it. Decide how you want to decorate your belly cast. How are you feeling as a pregnant woman? How would you like to be feeling, perhaps? Calm, fiery, exuberant, simple? Do you have a symbol that expresses your feelings? Do you have a symbol expressing your connection with your baby?

What colors would you like to use? What do those colors symbolize to you? Bring awareness to your choices in adorning your cast. Even if you are simply doing whatever comes into your mind as you are decorating, be aware of what the feelings associated with the embellishments might be.

Some women choose to mosaic their belly cast. Draw the general idea of what you would like to mosaic on the belly first. A tile cutter is necessary to cut the tiles / glass / wine bottles / mirrors into suitable shapes. Use tile adhesive or mosaic adhesive to attach the mosaics to the cast. If you use clear or sand-blasted glass, you can color the tile adhesive with different colors of paint—poster, acrylic, PVA—before placing the glass tiles on the cast. Grout the entire belly cast once you have finished placing the mosaics.

Alternatively paint the cast with two to three coats of acrylic paint. Beads, shells, feathers, found objects can be added if they have meaning for you. Be careful to keep it fairly simple and in accordance with your vision for it.

Decide where and how you would like to display your cast. Hanging it on the wall, surrounded by a simple frame of some sort can make a striking sculpture.

LABOR

Chapter Five

" Some writers have observed that, for a woman, having a baby has a lot of parallels with making a baby: same hormones, same parts of the body, same sounds, and the same needs for feelings of safety and privacy. How would it be to attempt to make love in the conditions under which we expect women to give birth? "

— *Dr. Sarah J. Buckley, Australian MD* [86]

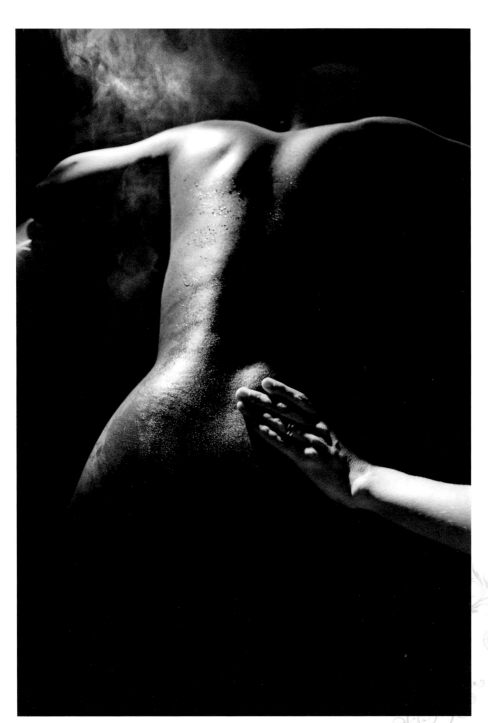

Signs of labor

If this is your first baby, or previous births have been artificially induced or been by Caesarean section, it can sometimes be difficult to distinguish between being in labor and being in the preparatory phase of labor. Giving birth is a natural process, that unfolds gradually. Your body and your baby will be preparing for birth weeks ahead of the actual labor.

Body preparations before birth

Braxton-Hicks surges: These surges usually become noticeable in the last trimester of pregnancy, although some women are aware of them earlier in the second trimester. They increase in intensity toward the end of the pregnancy, both in frequency and in intensity. Braxton-Hicks surges—named after the doctor who "discovered" them, although you can bet we women knew about them years before he did—are felt as a painless tightening of the uterus. Some women find that activity and becoming dehydrated can stimulate their occurrence.

The good thing to remember (especially if they are keeping you from sleep or focusing on tasks) is that they are preparing your body for true labor. They help to coordinate the uterine muscles to work efficiently when true labor begins and to soften (ripen) the cervix for progressive dilation in labor. Perceiving them as painful can be frustrating and tiring, as the expectation of entering true labor is so strong. It can become difficult to focus on the rest of your life if you are expecting to go into labor at any moment. Make sure you have a good deal of support if this happens to you, and remember that it is all positive preparation for the birth of your baby.

Engagement of the baby's head in your pelvis: This is also referred to as lightening, because as the baby descends into the pelvis, more space is created in your body above the womb. It is easier to breathe more freely, and you may experience less digestive discomforts, such as indigestion. Lightening sometimes only occurs at the start of labor, especially if you've given birth previously. If this is your first baby, it may occur two to three weeks before labor begins. The pelvic floor softens and becomes more relaxed. You may have to urinate more often and may have some numbness in your legs.

Backache: It comes and goes and feels similar to the backache of menstrual cramps. It can feel vague, low, and nagging and may cause restlessness.

Frequent soft bowel movements: This *may* be a sign of impending labor, if accompanied by other signs. It is a prostaglandin-induced change, which clears the lower digestive tract, making room for your baby's descent.

Energy spurt: This is sometimes referred to as a nesting urge, and you may feel yourself compelled to be active and busy. Save this extra energy for labor.

You may experience an increase in **Vaginal secretions.**

Weight loss: You may lose between half to one and a half kilograms (1.1 to 3 pounds). The changing levels of your hormones preparing for labor cause excretion of some of the extra fluid that accumulates during pregnancy.

Signs of pre-labor, which can alert you to birthing in the next day or two

A **"show"** of mucous mixed with some blood may be seen. It involves the mucous plug being expelled from the opening of the womb as your cervix begins to thin and soften in preparation for the birth. The mucous plug can release up to ten days before labor starts.

A **small rupture of membranes** causes a leakage of amniotic fluid from the vagina. It can sometimes be hard to tell whether you're having bladder leakage or amniotic leakage. A good way to tell is to void your bladder completely, then put on a menstrual pad, change positions/activity, and see if something leaks out. You may also want to note the color of the fluid. It should be clear and mostly colorless/odorless, not yellow or brownish or greenish. Check with your midwife or doctor if you are leaking amniotic fluid.

You may experience **intermittent surges** without an established pattern. These surges tend to be erratic. They may stop and start. They do not increase in intensity. They are usually not accompanied by backache. Walking and sleeping may cause them to stop for a while. These surges help to soften and thin the cervix, although they are unlikely to cause it to dilate in a first time mother. They may last as long as three to four minutes but are not regular.

It is almost impossible to sleep during true labor (although cases have been documented of women doing so); so if you can sleep, then make the most of it, as it will help to conserve energy for later.

Positive signs that active labor is beginning

These signs include **progressing surges** that have a regular pattern of occurrence. They last forty-five to ninety seconds and become stronger and closer together with time. They feel very strong and are noticeable in the abdomen, back, or in both. Remember that even though they are termed "contractions," they are contracting the top three-quarters of your uterus, while the cervix and lower quarter of your uterus expand and dilate. It can be helpful to visualize this during surges. The uterus becomes very hard during the surges. Henci Goer describes the difference between labor and pre-labor surges as follows: "You will feel them low in the groin or in the lower back. They may radiate from front to back or back to front or down your legs. They are dull and crampy like menstrual or gas cramps. Pre-labor contractions, which you may have been experiencing for months, feel like a tightening across your belly or like the baby suddenly stretched in all directions."[88]

If you are not staying home to birth your baby, you will probably want to go to the hospital or birth center when surges are regularly spaced, about five minutes apart and about forty-five seconds in length. Let them become established if this is your first baby. Once at the hospital your surges will be monitored, the status of your cervix checked, and your baby's heartbeat listened to. If you are not in true labor yet, you may be encouraged to go out to eat, take a long walk, or go home until things pick up.

If you are aware of **cervical cramping**, chances are it's the start of true labor, as the cervix is beginning to dilate. These sensations can feel like twinges deep inside the vagina; they are sharper and stickier than cramps, which are usually a more muscular sensation.

In active labor surges rarely exceed ninety seconds, whereas in pre-labor they may be as short as ten seconds or as long as ten minutes. In established labor they become longer and stronger as labor progresses. Remember, resisting the surges increases the intensity of the sensations you will be experiencing.

The **rupture of membranes** could result in a gush of amniotic fluid from the vagina. If this happens, it may be a sign that labor is about to start soon. You should contact your midwife or doctor and not take baths, have sex, douche, or insert tampons in your vagina, because any of these could increase the possibility of infection in the womb. If you have a gush rather than a slow leak of amniotic fluid, then usually labor will begin within twenty-four hours.

You will experience **a change in your state of consciousness**, becoming more inward as labor progresses, but usually you will be intensely aware of how everything and everybody "feels" at the start of labor. The pupils of your eyes may become dilated, and you may wish for the lights in the room to be lowered. You may also experience heightened alertness and sensitivity. Walking or squatting may increase the intensity of the surges during active labor, whereas changing your activity in pre-labor often diminishes them.

When you are in true labor, you would probably be having at least two to three surges in ten minutes, lasting over forty-five seconds each, accompanied by cervical dilation of three to four centimeters (1 to 1.5 inches). Often a good sign of labor progress is when you start to feel you need to be settled in one place and the surges are requiring all your focus. Follow your gut feeling. If you think you will be more comfortable in the place where you plan to give birth, and you feel that you need to settle in because things are really beginning to pick up, then its okay to go to hospital, even if they send you away. It can be very helpful to phone your caregiver and check with her on the phone first, too.

What to do at the beginning of labor

- Take a comfortably warm bath to relax yourself, if your membranes have not ruptured.
- Have a sleep if it's night time.
- Eat if you haven't eaten in several hours and it's your normal mealtime. Or have a snack accompanied by a large glass of water.
- Find a relaxing activity, to keep you from focusing on the surges. If you can focus on outward activities, you are unlikely to be in true labor yet, so need to conserve your energy as much as possible. Energy loss through anxiety and stress is very great, so enjoy the fact that your pregnancy will soon be ending, and that you will be meeting your baby soon.
- The process of moving from pre-labor into active labor can happen rapidly. Let your midwife or doctor know when things are starting to happen, so that they can arrange for your birth, and feel confident to call them at any time for confirmation of how you're progressing.

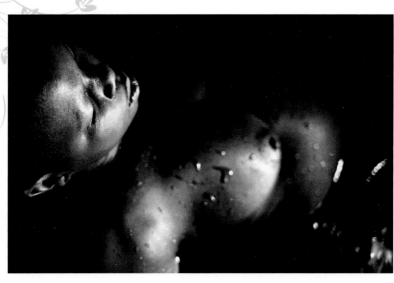

Opening to the sensations of labor

- Separate pain from fear. Find your natural coping style:
  Auditory: Use your voice. Make repetitive, mantra like sounds. Listen to music and relaxation tapes.
  Kinesthetic: Squeeze a pillow, get a massage, move around. Be aware of consciously relaxing your jaw, cervix, hands, brow, etcetera
  Visual: Use imagery, internal or external, for holding your focus through the surges.
- Use relaxation and visualization techniques.
- Use long, deep, letting-go breaths. Try out different breathing techniques before hand, and choose one that suits you.
- Let go into whatever you are experiencing without resistance. A study of meditators who were subjected to pain stimuli while connected to electroencephalographs (ECGs) found that they experienced only 10 percent of the intensity of the stimuli when they didn't resist and fight them.
- The use of focused awareness in labor is often a helpful technique for birthing women. Putting all your focus on something repetitive, which may be visual, auditory, kinesthetic, or imaginary, can act as a support during times when labor seems endless. Women are

naturally drawn to the places of repetition and focused awareness when they are deep inside their trance-like laboring space. The focus may be internal or external. The importance of focusing became so clear to me when Ulrike was laboring in a sunken Jacuzzi bath in a living area off her kitchen. Nearing the end of her labor, she was beginning to make the guttural birth noises that can help some women stay powerfully in their bodies at this time. I began to quietly draw the concertina doors between the kitchen and living area because her sleeping toddler's room was off the kitchen and I didn't want Ulrike worrying about waking her. "Don't do that!" she yelled. I stopped and looked at her. Her explanation was terse as if I could have intuited this and should have known better, "I'm watching the kettle!"

- Take one surge at a time.
- Make a noise, find your own sound—let sounds bubble up from deep inside. Make sure the sounds are low-pitched and powerful, let them come from deep down in your belly. Grunting, groaning, and bellowing can help some women let go. Don't scream, make high-pitched sounds, resistant sounds, or constrict your throat, as this only creates more tension.
- Singing or toning is a very empowering way to bring your body into a centered place where the energy is resonating in harmony with the surges.
- Dance. Belly dancing was originally designed for women in labor to free the pelvis and help them to open up. Dance helps one to enter the trance-like place of labor. It can create a special sense of intimacy with a partner if you dance together.
- Relax your pelvis and hips during each surge. Let them loosen, soften, widen.
- Hang by your arms from a rope, bar, or whatever is handy or set up. This allows your spine to stretch and is very relaxing.
- Walk, potter about, keep moving, especially in early labor. Keeping upright helps the baby to descend into the birth canal by gravity.
- Experiment with different positions—kneeling; kneeling with support; squatting; supported from behind by your partner; lying; leaning against a person, bed, or wall; sitting; sitting forward over a bed or bean bag. Do whatever helps or feels right.
- Exercise gently. Doing yoga stretches in labor can help relieve stress. If it hurts, then stop.
- There may be times in labor when you feel like moving, and other times when you want to rest
- Work with your baby.
- Labor support can be enormously beneficial, both from your partner or someone you

love, and also from someone calm who understands what you're going through and has been through labor herself. Focusing on and being deeply aware of support people can create a quiet, holding atmosphere, which encourages letting go.

- Touch and massage can be very soothing in labor. Feather-light strokes sometimes feel good on the belly, firm strokes often help on the lower back and over the hips, or down the legs. Some women dislike being touched in labor.
- Take baths/showers or use hot-water bottles. Water is very soothing in labor, although it may slow surges in early labor.
- Birth pools are often exactly what feel best in labor. You may choose to birth in the pool or get out after you are fully dilated. The reduced gravity can be especially helpful for backache during labor.
- Music, dimmed lights and aromatherapy may set up an atmosphere in a hospital labor ward. You may not be too aware of it if you're strongly focused on the labor, but it can send a helpful message to hospital staff to treat you quietly and calmly.
- If you aren't coping, you can always ask for pain relief. Using drugs in labor does not mean you've failed. They can have some side effects, though, especially in terms of disconnecting you from the experience of birthing. Be aware of that before hand, and then make your own decisions during labor.
- Labor is hard, sweaty, sometimes emotional, work. Disappointment can increase tension and intensify pain. Let go into exactly how your labor is for you, without setting up expectations for it to be perfect.

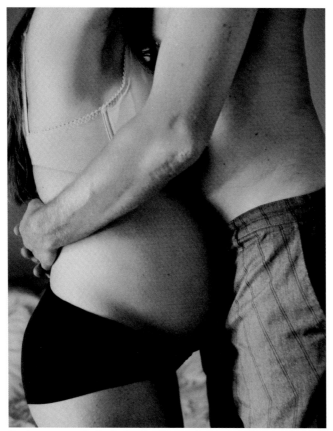

Partners are vitally important in assisting mothers to let go of resistance to labor.

Birth partners and fathers

" Speak tenderly to them. Let there be kindness in your face, in your eyes, in your smile, in the warmth of your greeting. Always have a cheerful smile. Don't only give your care, but give your heart as well. "

— *Mother Teresa, Nobel Peace Prize winner*

List of reminders for use with your partner during labor

- If labor begins at night and is light, help your partner back to sleep with a massage.
- If labor begins during the day, take her to a place you both love, where you can get used to labor together.
- Share a meal if she wishes to eat. She will need the extra energy later.
- Keep in close, relaxed physical contact with her.
- As labor progresses, help her to relax with any method that suits you both. For example, by encouraging her to let her body go limp between surges.
- Breathe softly and slowly with her if she starts to panic.
- Don't be embarrassed to use common endearments with the midwives around—your partner may need to hear them.
- You can act as intermediary between your partner and interested family and friends who call or come over or in some other way disturb the labor.
- As labor intensifies, your partner may find it helpful to use her voice. Encourage her to make noise if she needs to. Notice the pitch of her voice, and help her sounds be deep and guttural. High-pitched screaming sounds are indicative of resistance and fear. They build up more tension in everyone's bodies, and more pain in hers. Encourage her to continue making sounds, but to lower the pitch and to make sounds that are as deep as possible. Once labor has begun she'll only really "get it" if you show her by making the sounds yourself. It can help if you both practice beforehand.

When I was born, fathers were barred from attending births. Mothers were the primary caregivers, and my mother told me that my father hardly knew what to do with me in the first year. Only once I began toddling did he become a playmate. The presumption was that fathers didn't really know how to handle babies properly and it wasn't their job to do so. Gradually fathers were granted admission to be present in birthing rooms, and slowly they became more involved in baby rearing. Today, of course, parenting a baby is usually a task shared by both parents.

In this age of high Caesarean rates, partners sometimes request that they hold their babies while the mother is in post-operative care. Often these parents report that the partner has a closer rapport with their child than the mother does. No matter the type of delivery or birth method chosen, I encourage fathers to place their infant skin to skin against their chests for at least fifteen minutes within the first two to three hours of birth. The feedback is remarkable. Partners who have had previous children often report a much closer

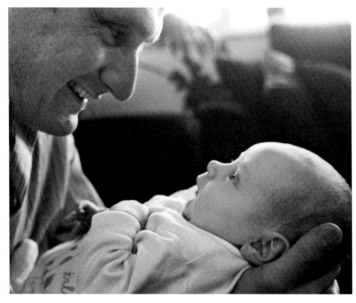

Fathers are given the opportunity to bond much earlier with their babies these days, often with life long benefits for their relationship. One advantage of Caesarean births is that they present an opportunity for fathers to develop a very early bond with their babies. This is improved with skin-to-skin contact and no disruptions.

relationship with their latest offspring, and usually they ascribe this to those early moments of bonding. Maybe it's the birth smell of our babies or the feel of their vernix and wet birth fluids against our skin that causes this initial attachment to occur—it defies rational explanation and has the feeling of instinctual and primary memories being stirred. It seems to occur not only in mothers, which we kind of expect, but in fathers, too.

Babies very clearly recognize both their parents at birth. I am trained to care for babies, and because I really like them, I expect them to respond positively to me. It is delightful to observe that babies far prefer their parents to me in the first hours after birth. When I pass a newborn from mother to her partner, they often tense slightly at my strange newness, and then wriggle into the comfort of this familiar person, who may never have touched them before.

In *The Secret Life of the Unborn Child*, Dr Thomas Verney refers to studies proving that babies recognize both parents' voices after birth.[90] He also mentions other studies that demonstrate how important it is for babies' and children's emotional well-being that they were exposed to a supportive relationship between their parents while in utero. Often the origins of childhood anxiety can be traced back to their mother's feelings of anxiety and insecurity—if there were consistent, deep levels of tension in her life during the pregnancy. The single biggest factor creating this type of tension was found to be her relationship with her partner.[91]

Verney refers to a trial involving more than 1,300 babies wherein those babies whose parents were undergoing relationship stress during the pregnancy were "five times more fearful and jumpy than the offspring of happy relationships." [92] However, thankfully, these effects are strongly ameliorated in babies who experience a strong sense of being loved by their mother.

Maternal hormones cross the placental barrier. A child whose life in utero was exposed to maternal hormones that signify happiness is far more content and self-assured than a child who was exposed to long-term production of stress hormones. Content babies have higher birth weights on average than anxious babies. Partners may think that they have a minor role to play in the healthy growing of their baby in the womb, but as these studies show, being a support person for their baby's mother is crucial for his or her well-being.

The Touch Research Institute at the University of Miami reports on a study demonstrating that fathers who gave their infants daily massages fifteen minutes prior to bedtime for one month showed more optimal interaction behavior with their infant.[93] Fathers are sometimes a little afraid of hands-on interaction with their newborns. Even today, some fathers feel that their partners have better parenting instincts than them. This can mean some fathers missing out on a really wonderful period of love and intimacy with their babies that is very different from the more social interactive relationship that develops later.

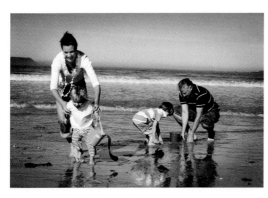

Sarah, Sebastian, Ollie, and Jono.

Sarah and Jono's birth stories

I asked Jono, Sarah's husband, to participate in the interview, so that we could have a partner's view of the birth process.

Oliver's birth

Oliver was born at home, in London, during a lunar eclipse. The midwife was off duty, her backup was off duty, and the third backup, whom Sarah and Jono had never met, arrived shortly before Ollie did. She had never attended a water birth, so Sarah had to get out of the birth pool. Sarah's mother, Sheila, who would have preferred a hospital birth, was the most experienced person there for most of the labor.

Jono: *Oliver's birth would have had to have drama in it. The types of birth were relevant. His birth was like his character, like he created his birth. The fact that there were two midwives who didn't show and a birth plan that didn't happen—even though the birth was beautiful and the environment intimate—it was still his stage and show. And there was a drama because the gas didn't work.*

Sarah: *The entonox gas for pain relief. It was an interesting introduction to parenting. The process of birth was so real, and the first reality was the loss of control. Everything was perfectly set up, and nothing worked according to plan.*

Jono: *For me, as an observer, my trust in the process was linked to my belief in Sarah and her clarity about how she wanted the birth to be. Her vision was very vivid for her—her preparation created a space which felt safe. Sarah was on track, and she had a willingness to go on this journey, which eventually went to the same destination, but with some detours. Selfishly we hadn't prepared for Sheila being there. Intimacy was something I wanted to share with Sarah. But actually, thank God, she was there!*

Sarah: *What was interesting for me since the birth was how many healing things from our childhood and our own births have happened. Mum often says my birth was tough. I can't remember the details, but I see that being at Oliver's birth was such a healing thing for Mum. It was absolutely healing for me too.*

Jono: *Being the only male present at the birth was hugely liberating for me. My perception of birth in our society had been that the medical professionals attending the births are often men. It felt like I hadn't handed over my intimate and privileged place to other men. From conception to birth, we start with intimacy and end with intimacy.*

Sarah: *A lot of people think we had a really bad birth with Ol. It was chaotic, but it was perfect, too.*

Jono: *I tell it with glee. For Ollie it would be an entertainment, like the actor he is—a story and a show. The time that Sarah was getting stitched and I was holding Ol—I still maintain today that that was when I really connected to him; he held my pinkie finger. I lay there exhausted and emotional, listening to Sarah in pain, and I remember feeling* >

it was so important that I could be there for him and how powerful that was for me.

Sarah: *The next day my original midwife arrived, and she showed us the extra entonox canister in the cupboard, so actually we had everything we needed for the birth.*

Jono: *Being at home was special. There was a familiarity with our environment, lying in our own bed, with our candles, our bath, our space; it felt safe and pretty significant and special. It was a lunar eclipse during Ol's birth, and I ran out into the overcast London night to try and video it.*

Sebastian's birth

Sebastian was born at home, in Cape Town , South Africa. Jono, Sue, and Robyn attended the birth. There was no time for Sarah to get into the birth pool.

Sarah: *The amazing thing about Sebastian's birth was how much I felt directed by connecting with him through the "unborn child" work we did. I felt really aware of who he was. That was kind of amazing; birthing someone you already know is a very different experience. Also the birth ceremony was so beautiful and also so right, and there was the whole incredible thing about the rainbows.* [The unborn Sebastian had requested a rainbow set of crystals. Then, seemingly unknowingly, many of the other participants in the birth ceremony brought rainbow gifts, and Sarah was given a beautiful rainbow-colored skirt to wear.] *After both births what really worked well for me was being in the water right afterward. Both babies and I really loved that.*

Jono: *After the birth, I felt hugely responsible with Ol. With Sebastian, though, I know he'll be okay. I'm more protective of Ol. I don't know if it's because of how they come into the world, or if it's that Ol is such a beautiful, sensitive soul.*

Sarah: *It was like Sebastian is really solid. There wasn't any drama. And he's not a dramatic child. We enjoyed it. He's such a contented baby and it was such a contented birth.*

Jono: *He smiled at me when he was born… thirty seconds after he was born. At the foot of the bed. When he came up onto Sarah's tummy, he looked up at me and he smiled. There's something around Sebastian's birth that's very interesting for me. I didn't feel separate from Sarah during Sebastian's birth. I felt like an observer at Ol's birth. I was a participant with Sarah; it was kind of erotic—primitive and sweaty, with Sarah grinding her head into my shoulder. It was so intimate. I was very relaxed, and we were with people who knew what they were doing and could hold the space for us. The last bit, the transition was so hectic yet intimate, and then there was suddenly* *this complete serenity. Sarah could breathe, Sebastian was relaxed, the crowning was slower. I found a space and relaxed into the process, in a way I never did with Ol's birth.*

Sarah: *There was a huge amount of relief. The intensity of both births being so fast and so intense, it was never something I was passively involved in: I birthed those babies. My involvement created the magic of the birth for me. It's that thing of duality— the intensity of the birth made the intensity of the pleasure afterward more extreme. There needs to be this process…*

Jono: *Rite of passage…*

Sarah: *A bridge—coming from one world into another world. Without that, it's too hectic. Kind of like, these days you can travel to places so quickly, it's disorienting. I can only imagine how it would be with an epidural or Caesarean. I feel you need the bridge of the intense birth experience. Transition is a good word for the hectic time. You are between two worlds. You emerge a completely new person when you've birthed a baby. You will never be the same person you were before you made that journey. It equips you the same way a journey in the external world can. The El Camino for instance—you emerge a different person after walking a pilgrimage route. Birth is like a spiritual journey. I bridged changes on all levels. Physically, I changed completely. Mentally, I worked through overcoming obstacles and fears. Emotionally, there's no more intense emotion you can feel. And spiritually, you are creating at the most profound level.*

Induction

Attending births is like growing roses. You have to marvel at the ones that just open up and bloom at the first kiss of the sun, but you wouldn't dream of pulling open the petals of the tightly closed buds and forcing them to blossom to your time-line.

— *Gloria Lemay, midwife and mother*

You may like to find out from your caregiver what percentage of their clients' vaginal births are induced or augmented? Induction and augmentation usually require epidural pain relief and the main reasons for doing them are convenience for you, the hospital, and the staff. If you have no sign of infection and are not a high-risk client, you probably wouldn't benefit from an induction or augmentation.

If your caregiver induces or augments most of their clients' vaginal births, they probably don't believe that the atmosphere in labor is important. Due dates are so variable. Some 5 percent of women give birth on their estimated date of delivery. First-born babies are more likely to go beyond their due date. Remember, too, that these dates are an estimation only. Babies generally know quite well when they are ready to come. If dates are inaccurate, babies who are induced may, in fact, be born prematurely.

Forty weeks from our last menstrual period is traditionally quoted as the expected due date for our babies. "Term" is defined as the time a baby is expected to be ready for birth. It refers to anytime between thirty-eight and forty-two weeks. In fact the average age of babies born without induction to first-time mothers has been found to be forty-one weeks and one day; if mothers have birthed previously, it is forty weeks and three days. Babies who are born earlier than thirty-eight weeks are considered premature, while those born after forty-two weeks have an increasing risk of receiving less than adequate nourishment from their mother's placenta, especially if they are smaller than usual for their gestational age.

In South Africa, women are often induced a week after their due date as an absolute cut-off point, or if they have no reservations about inductions, then on their due date. Some women are induced for convenience a week or two before their due dates. It is difficult for a neonatologist to accurately determine the weight of a baby within five hundred grams (1 pound) of his actual weight in utero. Babies are usually the right size for the pelvis, and when they start getting too big to fit, they come out.

A baby might seem too big if the mother is birthing with an epidural and lying in a reclining position, because then the power of her birthing muscles is reduced and the size of the pelvic opening is reduced. The size of the pelvis is not a very accurate indication of how easy it will be to birth. More important is the interior shape of the pelvis, which is difficult to estimate and which can change during labor anyway.

The biggest impediment to an easy descent through the birth canal for your baby seems to be when its head is incorrectly positioned for birth. This is more likely to happen if birth is induced or your waters have been artificially ruptured, as your baby may not have had time to get into the best position for birth yet. I have seen many babies over 4 kg (8.8 pounds) and up to 5.4 kg (11.9 pounds) birth easily given support, good birth positions, and patience.

Some 6 to 19 percent of women's amniotic sacs break before their labor has begun. Of these women, 90 to 95 percent will go into labor naturally within forty-eight hours without intervention. In the United Kingdom, according to the Royal College of Obstetricians and Gynecologists (RCOG) guidelines, women should be given the option of induction or expectant management with daily monitoring not exceeding 96 hours following membrane rupture.[94] If your waters break prior to labor, the following precautions will greatly minimize the risk of infection:

• Do not bath or sit in water.
• Do not insert anything into your vagina.
• Do not have vaginal examinations unless absolutely necessary.
• Maintain really good hygiene and wash your hands prior to and after using the toilet.

From a baby's perspective, inductions and augmentations that are not medically indicated are rarely helpful. The surges are more frequent and stronger than in natural birth. Less oxygen is delivered to the baby because the uterus has less time to become perfused with blood between the surges. The baby often experiences fetal distress, and then other interventions, like Caesareans, need to be introduced to manage the distress. If his mother chooses an epidural to cope with the pain of the increasingly severe surges, the baby doesn't experience relief. He will still be oxygen deprived, and he is more likely to feel dissociated from his mother and feel as if he is birthing all on his own, since his mother may have emotionally distanced herself from the birth after she became physically numb from the epidural.

Technique for inducing labor with a Foley's catheter

There is a method to assist women to begin laboring if they have gone way past their due date that is extremely simple yet effective, and which does not interfere with the normal course of labor in the way that drug-induced induction techniques do.

I learned it from a German obstetrician at the mission hospital in Botswana where I worked for a couple of years.

Your obstetrician or midwife will need to do this for you

A Foley's catheter, which can hold forty milliliters of water, is inserted into the cervix using a speculum and a sterile field. The balloon, which usually holds the catheter in place in the bladder, is then expanded in the middle of the cervix with forty milliliters (1.35 ounces) of sterile water and is left in place for up to six hours. Usually if the cervix is ripe, this stimulates enough production of prostaglandins for surges to begin, at which stage the catheter drops out as the cervix begins to dilate. If labor doesn't start after six hours, withdraw the water and remove the catheter. Pregnancy can then progress as normal or other methods of induction can be administered.

I suggested that my friend Jenny ask her obstetrician if he would use this method instead of a more interventionist method of induction, as she was two weeks past her due date and he wasn't keen to allow her pregnancy to continue for longer than that. She described the Foley's catheter technique to him and asked if he had heard about it. "Pft," he dismissed it with a shrug, "peasant technique." So instead Jenny was induced with misoprostol, a popular and particularly violent induction agent used by obstetricians in the United States and South Africa, and which often causes hypertonic surges and has been associated with rupture of the uterus. Jenny had a two-hour precipitated labor that was intensely painful and traumatic for her, and possibly for her daughter, too.

> Pregnancy is forty weeks at term –
> your baby will NEVER be easier to take care of than it is right
> there inside of you. Don't rush it!

— *Unknown*

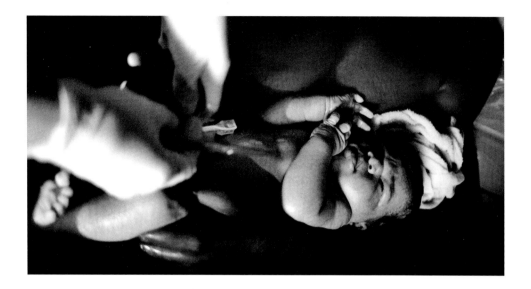

> Another thing very injurious to the child is the tying and cutting of the navel string too soon, which should always be left till the child has not only repeatedly breathed but till all pulsation in the cord ceases. As otherwise the child is much weaker than it ought to be, a portion of the blood being left in the placenta, which ought to have been in the child.
>
> — *Erasmus Darwin, Charles Darwin's grandfather, 1731-1802*[95]

Umbilical cord clamping

Minimal interventions at the time of birth make physiological sense to me. Our medical system, supported by our legal processes, sometimes seems to operate under the notion that unless proven otherwise, the more we control birth the safer it will become. If this erroneous principle were true, neonatal mortality rates would be significantly better in the countries with high rates of intervention like the United States (6.43 per 1000 live births = 36th best) and worse in countries promoting non-interventionist birth such as Sweden (2.76 per 1000 live births = 2nd best).[96]

The time of birth is a massive transition for a baby, moving from fetal circulation, to neo-natal circulation and from still being almost a part of his mother to becoming a separate, living, breathing being. He has been receiving his oxygen, nutrients, and mother's hormones from the placenta via the umbilical cord while in the womb. At birth, the umbilical cord continues to feed oxygenated blood to him for about five minutes until pulsation stops, while he gradually adapts to his surroundings, switches off his fetal circulation, and begins to breathe through his lungs.

In the first minutes after birth, particularly in a Caesarean-sectioned bab—which hasn't been squeezed through the birth canal—the lungs are still full of fluid. This fluid takes a short while to be fully absorbed into his system. If the baby is left undisturbed, he can slowly adapt to his new method of receiving oxygen via the breath while gradually letting go of his reliance on his mother's blood as a life-giving force.

Early cord clamping happens in the majority of births in Cape Town. In the Midwife Obstetric Units, clinics, and government hospitals, staff shortages require that the midwife or doctor completes the work involved in delivery as speedily as possible since there may be another woman with her baby's head already inching through her perineum next door.

Private practitioners seem to follow a similar trend. A childbirth educator reported to me that, at her antenatal classes' request, she phoned ten obstetricians in private practice to find out their protocols for cord clamping. Somebody in the antenatal class had heard or read about the theory that late clamping was beneficial for babies. This had instigated a request to find out what current practices in Cape Town were and to try to establish if indeed it was beneficial to delay cord clamping. All the obstetricians that were contacted cut the cord immediately after the baby was born.

After collating twenty-seven studies published in medical journals over the past forty years, gynecologist George Morley found that babies had higher hematocrits (and blood volume) if the umbilical cord is not cut immediately after birth. After birth, the newborn receives a transfusion of a third of its blood volume from the placenta if the cord is left uncut.

He concludes that, "Normal blood volume is not produced by a cord clamp. The newborn and placenta reach physiologic, hemodynamic equilibrium without interference. The placental transfusion is massive, silent, and invisible, but as normal and physiologic as is crying at birth. An adequate blood volume is needed to perfuse the lungs, gut, kidneys, and skin that replace the placenta's respiratory, alimentary, excretory, and thermal functions. During the third stage of labor, a large portion of placental blood is shifted to these organs. While the normal, term child tolerates immediate clamping, lack of placental transfusion

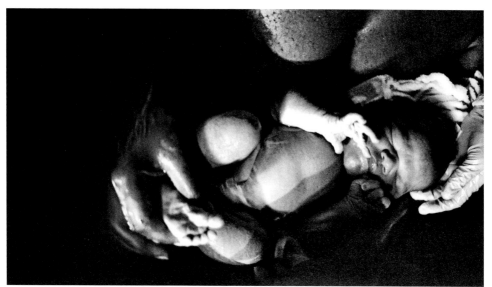

A baby whose cord is clamped after it has stopped pulsating, rather than at the moment of birth, is less shocked by the transition to extra-uterine breathing.

increases morbidity in "at risk" births. Many neonatal morbidities such as the hyperviscosity syndrome, infant respiratory distress syndrome, anemia, and hypovolemia correlate with early clamping. To avoid injury in all deliveries, especially those of neonates at risk, the cord should not be clamped until placental transfusion is complete."[97]

The increase in blood volume from the placenta if the cord is not cut immediately can cause a higher percentage of babies to develop physiological jaundice after birth, as their livers need to process fetal blood so that it adapts to neonatal circulation. We have learned to be afraid of jaundice after birth; however, the dangerous form of jaundice is pathological jaundice caused by blood disorders such as hemophilia. Physiological jaundice is rarely problematic, and if it does need treatment, babies can be placed under ultraviolet lights to help them develop Vitamin D to process the bilirubin. These lights can be rented so that the baby doesn't need to stay in hospital for the procedure. Milder forms of jaundice can easily be treated by undressing your baby and letting him lie in the sun for ten minutes twice a day. Choose a time of day when he will not be burned by sun exposure.

Many of the studies done around timing for umbilical cord clamping were undertaken between the 1960s and the 1980s. Interest waned thereafter, not because it was firmly established that early cord clamping was beneficial to babies—quite the opposite was established in the studies—but because interest seemed to decline in the issue when obstetricians handed over newborn care at birth to pediatricians. The pediatrician's job was to resuscitate the babies that were already presented to them at the resuscitation table, newly clamped and removed from the life-giving supply of oxygenated blood supplied by their mother's placenta. Since an obstetrician is already involved with the mother, he or she is more likely to view them as a unit. But, if a pediatrician is attending to the baby, it is understandable they would find it easier to work away from the mother, unimpeded by her fears that her baby is struggling for oxygen.

Recently, interest has arisen around the issue of cord clamping again. A study published by Kees Ultee et al in February 2007 looked at delayed cord clamping in pre-term infants delivered at thirty-four to thirty-six weeks gestation. The aim of the study was to provide neonatal and follow-up data concerning the effects of early or delayed clamping of the cord. The conclusion was that immediate clamping of the umbilical cord should be discouraged.[98]

Early cord clamping began when women were anesthetized during labor and at birth with ether. It is likely that the purpose of clamping the cord immediately was to minimize the amount of anaesthetic that was passing thorough the placenta to the infant. However, they were also depriving the infant of blood that rightly belonged to them, iron stores for the months ahead, and oxygen while they were adapting to breathing through their lungs.

Recently, it has become widely known that umbilical cord blood is rich in stem cells and that they can be harvested and used to restore bone marrow in deficient children. It's a lot cheaper and easier to just slow down birth and allow the child to absorb those rich, healthy stem cells while they're fresh and available, immediately after birth.[99]

The World Health Organization (WHO) no longer advocates early cord-cutting. According to the Royal College of Obstetricians and Gynecologists, there are no guidelines in this regard in the United Kingdom.

What does immediate clamping mean in terms of emotional trauma for the child? I can only report anecdotally here that I am saddened when I see a baby gasp as its cord is cut. The gasp is accompanied by a look of shock and by crying. Both reactions are unlikely to occur in a baby who has been given time to adjust to her surroundings before she begins to breathe of her own volition.

French obstetrician Frederick Leboyer, author of a revolutionary book called *Birth without Violence*, first published in France in 1974, was one of the first to call attention to our attitudes to our newborn babies, and to describe how susceptible newborns are to their environment. After describing the horrific scenario found at a "normal" hospital birth in the 1970s, he goes on to describe the alternative:

Learn to respect this sacred moment of birth,
as fragile, as fleeting, as elusive as dawn.
The child is there, hesitant, tentative,

Let him be.
Just wait.
This child is awakening
for the very first time.

This is his first dawn.
Allow him its grandeur, its majesty.
Don't even stir until he leaves behind
the night and its kingdom of dreams.

— *Frederick Leboyer, French obstetrician* [100]

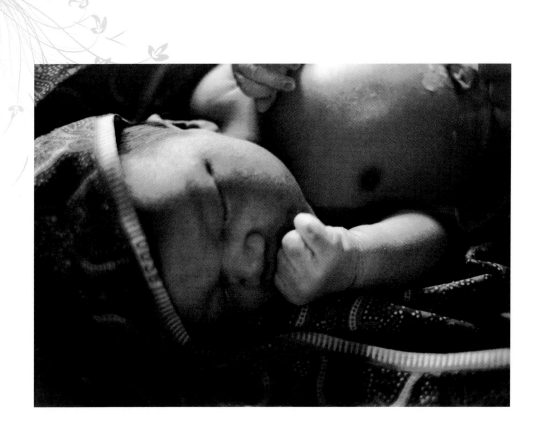

What is normal birth?

"

The question is disarmingly simple, like asking, 'What is love?'
I open my mouth to answer quickly, then close it again, suddenly
humbled by the realization that the answer is complex, emotional,
elusive, rich, deep, and varied.

Images flash in my mind—I see beautiful, wet babies in their
mothers' arms, I smell the birth smell and feel the holiness that
hangs in the air; and I feel the wonder that rises in the presence
of the wise and ancient process that is beyond human design or
control.

Normal birth is the mother who stands up beside her bed where she has just given birth, faces me with her babe in arms, her eyes flashing fire and triumphantly shouts, 'I did it!'

Normal birth is the woman who dances the slow birth dance and sings the low birth song. It is the woman who is naked and not ashamed.

Normal birth is the woman who, though she has never been there before and did not know she knew the way, finds her path to the deep and quiet place within herself where her intuition and faith lie hidden and ready to feed her soul.

Normal birth is the woman who births in her own power, dignity, beauty, grace, and strength. It is this mother and this never-seen-before baby working it out together for the first time.

Normal birth is what I trust this mother can do, it is what I believe in, cherish, and humbly protect. It is the gift we give the mothers we serve and the gift they give their precious babies. It is the real-life miracle I witness again and again with an ever-growing sense of privilege and joy.

— *Lois Wilson, American midwife*[101]

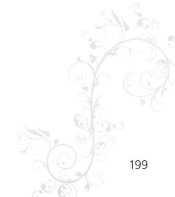

Immediately after birth

To a mind that is still, the whole universe surrenders.

— *Chuang-tzu, Taoist philosopher, 4th century BCE* [102]

Labor is hard work for your baby. In regression work performed in the Sixties using LSD, Dr Stanislav Grof found that babies experienced their births as a process of being painfully squeezed through a very tight and constricted space. At birth, she is suddenly free of the constriction and her senses are flooded with new impressions and feelings. Even if she had a birth without interventions, which would have been easier for her to cope with, she still needs time to adjust to the newness of her strange environment without disturbance if she is not to contract in shock. She needs quiet—the quietness that comes from recognizing the sacredness of the experience for her. Anything that reminds her of the womb, so that she can relate to that which she already knows, will be soothing to her. Your voice, your hands, your partner's touch, warm water, appreciation, and gentleness will help to settle her. Don't rush her; this moment of birth is enchanting. Open your heart to its timelessness as fully as you can.

Babies also need to be kept warm after birth. Michel Odent, French doctor and midwife, claims that a heater is the most important item in a midwife's birth kit. The best place to keep your baby warm is on your chest, skin to skin, and covered by a warmed towel or blanket. The birth room should be warm enough and free from draughts. Breast-feeding within an hour of birth provides your baby with calories to produce body heat.

Her most significant need at this time is for love. This is her first impression of life. What she learns at the moment of birth will stay with her. Love will teach her that she can trust life. Even if you are separated for any reason, send her love using mental imagery. She'll get it, and it will be the most important piece of her birthing history.

The placenta

Sometime in the initial period after birth, the placenta will deliver. Your options are to deliver it yourself with a few, usually mild surges, or with the assistance of the caregiver who tugs at it during a surge to help it birth.

Sometimes, parents decide not to discard the placenta, since it is seen in various cultures to hold symbolic significance itself. As it was responsible for nourishing the baby for so many months, it is seen symbolically as the nurturer.

In Ayurvedic traditions, it is believed that the placenta connects the consciousness of the child in the womb to his divine essence. This has led to a practice in the East called "lotus birth," where the placenta is left attached to the cord and the baby until the cord spontaneously drops off at the baby's umbilicus. In many other traditions, the placenta is buried; sometimes, it is planted under a tree, so that the tree can draw nourishment from it as it degenerates. The placenta needs to be buried deep in the ground, since it could be too nutrient rich for a sapling if the roots touch it immediately.

Often this is accompanied by a short ceremony. Sometimes, the ceremony occurs at the same time as the baby naming. The tree then belongs to the baby, and if water is used during the blessing of the baby to anoint it, the remainder of the water can be sprinkled over the roots of the tree.

AFTER BIRTH

Chapter Six

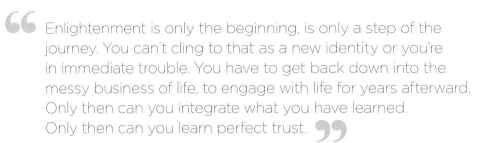

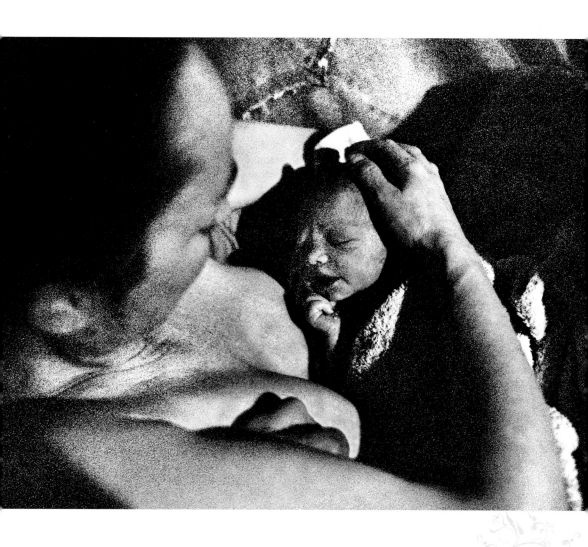

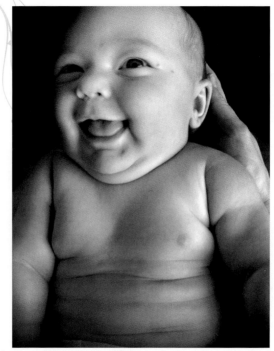

Lots of attention, time, and acceptance of things being okay, despite being tiring, can help our babies settle into their beautiful bodies.

Like enlightenment, birth is simply a stepping stone to a new way of living. Giving birth to the most perfect baby, in the most empowered way, doesn't change the fact that we have diapers to wash and hours of sleep to catch up on, although it often does provide the satisfaction of knowing we can do anything, even this.

Clare was coming toward the end of her pregnancy. It was, in fact, the day before she gave birth, and she had realized how loath she was to let go of her time of growing and being so intimately connected to her baby. Her pregnancy was awe-inspiring—deeply connected to her body and her baby, she had developed that aura of wholeness that is supposed to radiate from pregnant women. Clare wondered whether baby blues were a period of mourning for the loss of this special time. The following day she went into labor, and for a while after birth everything seemed to unravel in a way over which she had no control.

Some women fly on a creative high for up to a year after the birth of their baby while others become confused and overwhelmed; some seem to experience a combination of both states. They seesaw between highs and lows, feeling like they're losing control, so vulnerable are they to their ever-changing emotional state. Sometimes we feel like we're blossoming in a wonderful creative bloom after birth, at other times we can feel as if we're imploding.

Nobody seems to have any real answers to how to avoid the low periods, or even any real understanding of how the same woman could have tremendously different experiences after the births of each of her babies.

We seem to take the normal surge and expansion of our creative life force and crank it into psychedelic overdrive after birthing babies. The cycles of life expand outward and contract inward in a rhythmic flow of yin and yang. Both are equally important. We like the expansion because it's productive and exuberant. We often try to avoid the contraction because we are taking what we learned during the expansive phase and reflecting on how it affected us. Very often these quieter periods cause feelings of judgment and self-criticism to arise.

Some women view pregnancy as enormously creative—growing the baby and growing a connection to him that will last a lifetime. Some women see birth as the final outburst of this creative act (and others choose to avoid the intensity of birth at all costs). Some women identify most closely with their newborn during interactions and begin a whole new love relationship, so to them this becomes the more creative and satisfying portion of the birth experience. Some women don't get their creative kicks from babies much at all. All of us, however, are required by our bodies to follow the cyclic rhythm of creative, expansive periods followed by quiet times of reflection.

The women who adapt best to motherhood aren't always on a high. They may mourn the loss of their pregnancies and cry quite freely, fairly often, and for various reasons. They usually stay connected to their babies, patiently recognizing the spirituality of the process without judging their abilities as women and mothers. They take time to be quietly by themselves, too.

As Eicho wrote in a Japanese haiku poem many years ago,

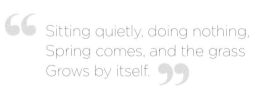

Sitting quietly, doing nothing,
Spring comes, and the grass
Grows by itself.

— *Eicho* [104]

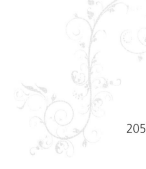

Taking care of yourself

> Besides the noble art of getting things done, there is a nobler art of leaving things undone. The wisdom of life consists in the elimination of non-essentials.

— *Lin Yutang, Chinese writer and Nobel Prize nominee*

- If you feel okay, then your baby will relax and enjoy life more.
- Your own needs are as important as your baby's needs.
- You'll get all the advice you need, and more, from friends, caregivers, and relatives. Choose what suits your mothering style best after investigating all the options.
- Eat healthily and keep physically active.
- Allow for disruptive pregnancy hormones.
- Lower your expectations.
- Be easy on yourself.
- Let go of your need for your baby to behave in a certain way or sleep better than he does; you can't control it.
- Be patient with bonding and breast-feeding.
- Life isn't perfect, so remember once again: *be easy on yourself.*

Kangaroo care

Kangaroo care is the term used to describe skin-to-skin swaddling of mothers with their babies. It is a method of incubating babies on their mother's chests to keep them warm and to stabilize their heartbeats and breathing. Clinical trials on premature babies have found that it also helps babies sleep for longer periods, gain weight faster, increase their brain development, and improve breast-feeding. As a result they have less periods of "purposeless" activity, which uses up precious energy reserves, and longer periods of alertness. In comparison with premature babies who are cared for solely in incubators, they are generally discharged from hospital sooner.

The method requires that your baby be dressed only in a diaper and a warm cap. He is placed chest to chest in direct skin-to-skin contact between your breasts. The direction his head is facing should be changed after every feed. Together with your baby, you are

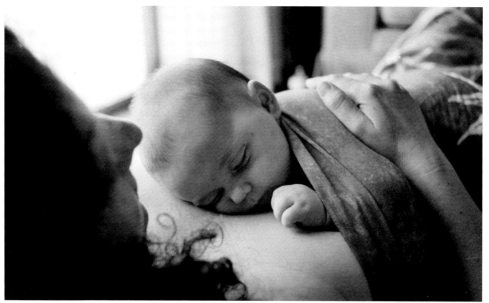

Kangaroo care nurtures the parent-infant bond and is beneficial for all babies.

then wrapped in a receiving or swaddling blanket so that you are bound close together. A warmer outer blanket can cover your baby in cooler weather.

Tiny babies are unable to regulate their body heat well and their temperature can drop fast if they are exposed to draughts and cool air. However, as mothers, we have an extraordinary mechanism in our bodies for regulating our infant's temperatures. Your skin temperature will increase by at least 2°C on the side of your body that he is lying against if his body temperature is low. If he is moved to the other side of your chest, within two minutes your temperature will have increased by at least 2°C on that side and dropped on the side that he left. Conversely if he is too warm, your skin temperature will drop to bring him back into homeostasis.

If your baby is kept close to your breasts, he will feed more easily and more strongly than babies who sleep separately from their mothers. It is only necessary to loosen the swaddling blanket slightly to latch your baby; he does not need to be removed from his "kangaroo pouch" for feeding.

Kangaroo care research has largely been undertaken with premature babies. It has been consistently proven that babies thrive better when swaddled with their mothers than when isolated in an incubator.[105] This research doesn't only have implications for premature babies; all babies benefit from kangaroo care. Most parents find that kangarooing their baby for two to three hours

207

a day is an experience they later treasure as having created the most beautiful bonding. Krisanne Larimer writes about her feelings about kangarooing her premature infant in an online article on kangaroo care benefits: "Holding that tiny body next to mine, feeling her little hand clutching my collar bone, feeling her drift to sleep in my arms... truly the most amazing experience of my life."[106] This feeling of contentment is mirrored in the babies as well. Measurements of their brain-wave patterns during kangaroo care show a doubling of alpha brainwaves, which are associated with states of bliss and feelings of well-being.

In the days following birth, hypothermia, or low body temperature, can be prevented by keeping the baby and mother together (rooming-in), by breast-feeding as long and as often as your baby wants, and by dressing your baby appropriately for the environmental temperature.

In a Swedish study of eighty hypothermic newborns, forty were placed in incubators and forty were held skin-to-skin by their mothers. After four hours, 90 percent of the infants who had skin-to-skin contact had reached a normal body temperature while only 60 percent of the infants placed in incubators had done so. After twenty-four hours, the body temperatures of the incubated infants were slightly higher than those of the held infants, suggesting that incubated infants run a risk of becoming too warm and developing heat stress. Skin-to-skin contact also stabilizes heart and respiratory functions, according to the researchers.[107]

The Touch Research Institute in Miami found that pre-term infants who received tactile stimulation showed greater weight gain. A potential underlying mechanism for the massage/weight gain relationship is an increase in vagal tone, which in turn increases food absorption.[108]

There is an assumption in the medical world that a baby requires incubator care in order to stabilize. In a randomized controlled trial conducted by Bergman et al, it is stated that "The reality is that incubators actually 'de-stabilize' newborns. Newborns have a brain-wiring (neurophysiology) that craves and requires mother's presence in order to stabilize, in order to achieve adjustment to a new environment and physiological homeostasis.... Newborn care provided by skin-to-skin contact on the mother's chest results in better physiological outcomes and stability than the same care provided in closed servo-controlled incubators. The cardio-respiratory instability seen in separated infants in the first six hours is consistent with mammalian 'protest-despair' biology, and with 'hyper-arousal and dissociation' response patterns described in human infants: Newborns should not be separated from their mothers."[109]

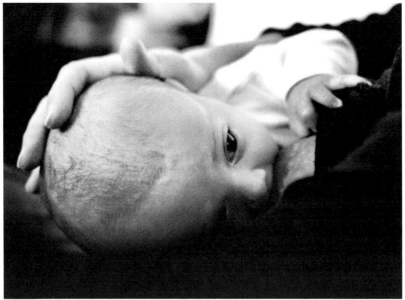

Giving your baby love when you are breast-feeding is as nourishing emotionally as breast milk is nourishing physically.

Breast-feeding

Breast-feeding is fairly simple when you know how.

" When we trust the makers of baby formula more than we do our own ability to nourish our babies, we lose a chance to claim an aspect of our power as women. Thinking that baby formula is as good as breast milk is believing that thirty years of technology is superior to three million years of nature's evolution. Countless women have regained trust in their bodies through nursing their children, even if they weren't sure at first that they could do it. It is an act of female power, and I think of it as feminism in its purest form. "

— *Dr Christiane Northrup, Specialist in women's health issues* [110]

— Dr Frank Oski, Retired editor, Journal of Pediatrics[111]

To most women, breast-feeding sounds like a good idea. In Botswana, in the mission hospital I worked in, breast-feeding problems were relatively rare. If a new mother was confused about how to feed her baby, someone else in the ward or a midwife would quickly resolve problems with latching. Perhaps this was partly because, culturally, breast-feeding is the norm, partly because feeding is done in public, so everyone has some idea how it's done, and partly because the pace of life is slower in the rural areas where I was working.

In the West, unlike in many cultures, we are seldom exposed to breast-feeding education from our mothers, aunts, elder sisters, or extended family. To manage breast-feeding successfully in our culture, we sometimes need support, education, and encouragement. A lactation consultant can usually sort out initial feeding problems swiftly and effortlessly. Some hospitals have a lactation consultant on call, and if you birth at home many consultants are happy to pay you a home visit. Alternatively, you can ask your home-birth midwife for advice.

The idea of breast-feeding loses its appeal and may bring a grimace to the face of a mother struggling with cracked nipples or mastitis. Nevertheless, it offers so many advantages to maternal and infant well-being that one wonders why we struggle to manage it sometimes.

Colostrum, which is produced in the first few days, is full of antibodies, immunoglobulins, leukocytes, and easily digestible protein. It is thicker than milk, is a yellowish color, and is produced in droplets at a time. Do not worry if your baby doesn't seem to be getting much to drink. Colostrum is produced in very small quantities, is very nutritious, and provided she is latching well is all she needs for the first few days.

Between days three and five, your milk starts to increase in volume. If you are feeding your baby regularly, you will not experience this change dramatically as the baby regulates the milk supply. Most breast-feeding problems occur in the first six weeks, while both mother and baby are learning from one another.

Getting started

Start breast-feeding within two hours of birth if you can. Your baby has a particularly strong sucking and rooting reflex immediately after birth and it is a good time to initiate breast-feeding. The after-effects of epidurals can make a baby drowsy after birth, in which case, leaving baby skin-to-skin on your chest until your baby is ready to feed is highly recommended. Should your baby not latch, try expressing some colostrum onto a spoon and feed your baby with this regularly (every ten to twenty minutes) until he is ready to latch.

Latching

Latching your baby well is the key to managing breast-feeding without problems. Make sure you are comfortable and choose a position that suits you. The positions are described below.

Cradle your baby on your forearm facing you, making sure her tummy is against your body. Your nipple should be in line with her nostrils before latching. Support her head gently without pushing it against your breast. Tickle her lower lip with your nipple so that she opens her mouth in a rooting reflex. If she seems reluctant to open her mouth, express a little colostrum onto the nipple. This usually encourages the rooting reflex. When her mouth is wide open, draw her gently toward your breast. Try not to lean forward and bring your breast to her; this often causes babies to arch backward. She will far prefer it if you bring her to the breast. Watch her lower lip, and aim it as far down over the lower areola as possible, so that her tongue draws a large portion of the areola into her mouth. There should be more of the lower than upper areola in her mouth. If she is only attached to your nipple, it will hurt, she won't be able to get much milk from the breast and eventually it will lead to blisters and cracked nipples. A good latch depends upon her attaching to your areola rather than your nipple, as this is where the ducts that release the milk are situated. Breathe deeply, and focus on relaxing and settle into allowing her to feed for just as long as it takes. When she is full, she will usually drop off. If you have to take her off for any reason, and it is preferable that you do not, release the latch by inserting your finger into the corner of her mouth.

Try to avoid forcing her to your breast, pulling her chin down to open her mouth, or flexing her head as you bring her to your breast. It is helpful to cup your breast with one hand, hold it still, and guide your baby to the breast with the other. Don't move her onto the breast before she has opened her mouth.

Find the position most comfortable for you and your baby. Vary positions until you find one that works because different positions may help with better latching.

- **The cradle hold** is the traditional position with your baby resting on your forearm. You can then bring her to the breast by moving your arm closer to your body.
- **The cross cradle hold** is similar to the cradle hold but you switch arms.
- **The football hold** is the term for tucking her under your arm with her legs wrapped around your body and facing backward.

- **A maternal side-lying position**, with your baby lying alongside you, is useful to initiate breast-feeding directly after Caesarean birth and when you are sleeping.

The milk ejection reflex (MER), or let-down reflex, is increased with rest, relaxation, and a comfortable position. This can be felt by some mothers as a tingling feeling in the breast and the other breast starts to leak. If you cannot feel this, do not be concerned so long as your baby is satisfied after each feed and gains weight adequately. It is okay to let your baby spend the entire feed on just one breast to ensure that she gets the benefit of the richer hind-milk that is produced toward the end of a feed by each breast. If she is properly latched, it will not be a problem for your nipples. You can alternate breasts during a feed if she looks like she wants both breasts, but offer one breast until she comes off the breast satisfied. Babies cannot tell time; therefore, timing at the breasts is totally unnecessary.

Be patient with yourself, this is a learning experience for both of you, so without interference and with some belief in yourself you will get it right. Good maternal nutrition, rest, and relaxation time all help with establishing a healthy milk flow.

Feed on demand until she has settled. Demand feeding means beginning a feed when she is starting to move around, placing her hands near her mouth and starting to look awake, rather than when she is already crying. This is the time to feed her. If she is crying she usually will not latch easily as she will be too angry. To increase your milk supply you just need to allow your baby to feed whenever she wants to. In the initial few days she may want to suckle most of the time, or she may be tired from a long labor or drowsy from an epidural and not be that interested in feeding. During the first two weeks, wake her for feeds if she is sleeping for longer than two hours during the day, although you can allow one sleep of four hours in a twenty-four hour period if she is feeding well at other times. Once breast-feeding is established and she is more settled, the periods of sleep can extend to beyond this length of time.

Helpful breast-feeding tips

- Nipple pain: Prevent nipple and breast pain with good latching and frequent feeding. Start on the least painful side. Change breast pads often so that your nipples don't become too damp. Putting breast milk onto the nipples is the best nipple cream you can find. Break your baby's suction on your breast by inserting your finger into the side of her mouth, rather than pulling her off the breast.
- Engorgement: This can occur as the milk comes in but can be avoided by regular feeding from birth and by staying together with your baby to establish breast-feeding. Ice packs on the breasts between feeds will help relieve the swelling. Expressing the areola prior to feeding your

baby can be helpful to soften the nipple so that your baby can latch more easily. Remember that this is a transitory phase and clears most quickly if you keep feeding regularly.

- All babies are sometimes fretful for reasons that *no one* can understand. Try not to take it as a personal rejection. Babies always benefit from a calm, loving atmosphere. Move slowly, gently, quietly.
- Becoming aware of when your baby cries in relation to her feeding pattern is often a good way to assess her needs. Consider the following options if you are not sure why your baby is crying, but think she may be hungry:
  - If she's due for a feed and is fretful, try feeding her first to see if this is the problem. Remember babies cannot tell the time and, therefore, need to feed whenever they demand it. Sometimes they go through growth spurts, which can occur at six weeks and three, six, and nine months. They will suddenly seem to need more regular feeds; if you feed them on demand, these extra feeds will usually last for two to three days.
  - Some babies dislike having wet or soiled diapers more than others. If this seems to be causing the problem, change her first before feeding.
  - Is she too warm or too cold?
  - Is her clothing comfortable? Does she have any skin irritation?
  - Check that your baby is properly latched, with a large portion of the areola in her mouth. A poor latch will mean that she will be receiving less colostrum or milk and your nipples will become painful.
  - Your baby might be positioned uncomfortably. Make sure she is lying horizontally and that her neck is not at an angle. Be gentle with burping her. If the wind needs to come up, it does so best when you remain patient and let her relax gently against your shoulder or sit her upright on your lap. If she doesn't burp, maybe she doesn't need to. Thumping her on the back does not bring the wind out any easier; it only makes her more irritable. Just hold her gently and if the wind comes out, that's great, if she doesn't burp, then it's okay to place her down in bed. Remember that babies do not like to be separated from you in the first few weeks; often she may cry after being put down because of separation anxiety, not because of wind.
  - Is she overtired? Sometimes, the shortest nap can help soothe a fussy baby. Babies will often settle easily when they are placed skin-to-skin with you or your partner.
  - Are you overtired? Sometimes a short nap for yourself while someone else watches your baby can help soothe everyone, including the baby.
- Try taking a deep warm bath with your baby. The moist heat, holding her, and relaxing all help

- Burping up small quantities of half-digested, cheesy milk after feeds may be caused by a slow digestive system. This may occur when your baby is fussy or simply bringing up air with some food in front of it. Pathological vomiting, which needs medical attention, is characterized by projectile vomiting, extreme irritability, and subsequent failure to gain weight.
- Over stimulation can cause fussiness, especially if your baby is tired. Don't always have too many toys around her when she is awake. Watch for the cues of when she is interested in seeing objects around her and learn when she needs them taken away. Try to provide a calm atmosphere. If you know that a particular time of the day is difficult for your baby, try to get some rest yourself prior to that time so that you are calmer and more easygoing with her. Sometimes, she will have a daily need for a period of "cluster feeding." During this time, she will become more demanding than usual. It often coincides with a busy family time. It is a good idea to feed her more often when she is so fussy. Usually babies will cluster feed for a period of about four to six hours, feeding every half-hour. and then eventually will fall peacefully asleep. Although this may be difficult for you, especially if you have other children, it will pass. Having supper all prepared ahead of time, and perhaps having someone come and help at that time with the older children, is useful. It can also be helpful to have a sling in which you can place your baby or, to place her in the area where the family are all busy.
- Although it can be enormously frustrating to be given endless advice from overly helpful people, it can be helpful to let one person whom you trust teach you how to soothe your baby if you haven't had a baby before. They can also take the baby from you to give you some rest when you feel you aren't coping.

Contra indications to breast-feeding

There are occasionally times when it is best not to breast-feed your baby:
- If you are HIV+ you would be wise to formula-feed your baby whenever it is safely possible, to prevent the HIV virus passing through your breast milk. Some recent studies have shown that breast-feeding, without any supplementation from bottles or food for the first three to six months, doesn't significantly increase the transmission rate. However, the risk through breast-feeding is cumulative—and the longer an HIV-infected mother breast-feeds, the greater the risk of transmission to her baby. A review of available evidence has been collated by UNICEF, UNESCO, WHO, UNAIDS, and UNFPA, and a pdf file may be found on their Web site.
- If you are undergoing either chemotherapy or radiation treatment for cancer, you should avoid breast-feeding.

- If you are on medication, check with your doctor to ensure that it will not affect your baby. If you are taking recreational drugs or abusing alcohol, it's good to know that they do pass through your breast milk to your baby to a greater or lesser degree, depending on the substance.

How to tell if your baby is getting enough milk

- She has more than six wet diapers in twenty-four hours.
- She seems healthy.
- She gains between one hundred and fifty and two hundred grams (5.3 to 7 ounces) a week after the first week. (Breast-fed babies usually lose a little weight in the first couple of days).
- Do not worry about the number of stools your baby passes. Because breast milk is so well digested, your baby can go for a week without passing a stool if she is breast-fed.

When to take your baby to your health-care provider

Take your baby to your health-care provider to get her checked if:

- Her fontanel is sunken after a good feed.
- She has no wet diapers in a day.
- She is listless.
- Her skin is losing its elasticity, which is a sign of dehydration.
- She loses more than 5 percent of her weight.
- She doesn't gain weight weekly.

Weaning

When, why, and how to wean are important questions to ask. You do not have to fully wean your baby if you are returning to work. If you are lucky enough to have child care at work, then during your coffee and breaks times you can go to your baby and continue to fully breast-feed.

If you are going to be away from your baby during the day, you could express your breast milk while at work and transport it home. You will need sterile containers to express it into and a fridge or cooler filled with ice blocks in which to keep it cold. This milk will then be given to your baby the next day. If this is not an option, then a gradual approach to weaning is easiest. Start with one cup or bottle-feed replacing one breast-feed, adding another one after three days to a week, and so on until she is weaned. If you only need her

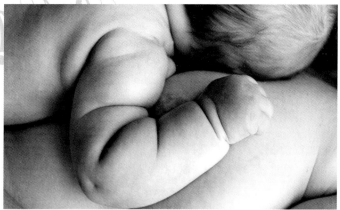

Breast-feeding is a time for relaxing, taking a few deep breaths, and settling into the moment.

to be weaned during the day, then you continue with the morning and evening feeds. It is very convenient and a wonderful way to say hello to your baby after a day at work to breast-feed as soon as you get home and to continue to breast-feed at night and in the morning until you leave for work.

Breast-feeding meditation

Breast-feeding is a time when your state of mind impacts significantly on your baby's state of consciousness and also quite likely, on the quantity and quality of your milk production.

Michel Odent, French obstetrician, endocrinologist, and an inspiration to many midwives worldwide, has done in-depth research on the emotional effects of various hormones. Oxytocin, he claims, is a "love" hormone, and when we produce oxytocin we feel surges of love, either for our partner (on orgasm) or for our babies (during birth or breast-feeding). Orgasm, labor and breast-feeding are the three times in our lives when we produce oxytocin in large quantities. Oxytocin causes the "let-down" reflex for breast-feeding mothers, which in turn creates the surge of milk shortly after the baby starts to suckle.

It follows, then, that if oxytocin creates a feeling of love to arise in us, if we focus on feeling love for our babies, and allow a surge of love to flow through us when we feed them, perhaps that will help the flow of oxytocin and increase our milk production. Hormones and the endocrine system are the physical expression of our emotional state of mind, and they truly do represent a very concrete example of the mind-body connection—the interdependence of mind and body. Michel Odent also states that a mother and baby gazing at each other after birth is instrumental in inducing the rush of oxytocin, which causes the uterus to contract effectively.

I have a completely unsubstantiated sense that if a mother's milk is drenched with love it may have physiological benefits for her child, and possibly could make a baby fatter and more content, with a stronger immune system.

Breast-feeding meditation

Here, then, is a meditation to help you relax and focus on your baby with love while breast-feeding:

This meditation can be useful for times of day when you know your baby is likely to feel stressed. Often our babies are uncomfortable at the end of the day, usually when we are feeling at our most tired, and when their siblings are also requiring lots of attention. A suggestion is to use this meditation for the feed prior to the one when your baby is often stressed, then make sure you take at least half an hour for yourself before the next feed, to simply relax and unwind. Alternatively, take time just to relax and do nothing else but enjoy your baby, and then use the meditation again at the time when feeding can be more difficult.

Even though it may seem as though there simply isn't enough time in the day to make space for yourself, it is well worth trying because, very often, if you are calm and relaxed enough, your baby may settle more easily as well, thus freeing you up to do all the other things that require your attention after the feed.

It may only be necessary to use this meditation a few times to get the idea. Thereafter, you could bring yourself into your own quiet and reflective state when you settle down to feed your child. Playing soothing music during feeds can help you both to settle, particularly if your baby responds well to music that was played to her in the womb. Use the advice on breast-feeding positions to help you latch your baby correctly: a good latch helps with milk production and with avoiding most breast-feeding problems.

To avoid your baby waking fretful and hungry prepare for the feed in advance. Make sure you have a glass of water on hand and a comfy feeding chair with cushions for adjusting your posture, so that you will both be comfortable.

Take a few minutes before your baby will need his feed to sit on your own, breathing deeply and relaxing yourself. Be aware of coming into the present moment. Feel >

the state of your body. Are there areas of your body that feel tired; is there anywhere that is holding discomfort or tension? Breathe deeply into these areas. Sense how you experience the tiredness, stress, or discomfort. Be aware of these states without offering any resistance, simply by opening up to how that feels.

Allowing a moment or two for yourself, bring a sense of tenderness into your body, into the places of tiredness or stress. Breathe into them with love, acknowledging that it is as important for your baby that you have compassion for yourself as it is for you to care deeply for them. Breathing in and out, slowly and deeply, simply take a few moments just for yourself. Breathe into your heart and allow this feeling of tenderness to seep from your heart all the way through your body, particularly into the places that have been feeling uncared for and neglected. Let your heart open in sympathy for any part of yourself that is not totally peaceful and calm.

Pause the meditation for a few moments to fetch your baby and prepare for feeding. Continue the meditation once you and your baby are ready to begin feeding and you are both comfortable. Take in another deep breath and breathe out love to your baby. Settle into this moment. Place any other thoughts and activities aside for this time and simply focus your awareness on your baby. Gaze into your little baby's face, and allow your feelings of love for your baby to flow through your breast milk into their body. Be aware of the softening and specialness of this moment.

Focus your awareness on the feelings of your baby suckling. Surrender into this moment. Simply remaining open to the pleasure of being with your baby and nourishing and nurturing her with love. If it feels appropriate touch your baby's skin with love, stroke, caress, and nurture her, sing lullabies to her, or simply sit with your baby in silence and hold a space of tranquility and peace for her to be fed within. As you become more serene and peaceful, breathing in calm and breathing out love to your baby, so you may find she responds with reciprocal behavior. Feel her soft yet focused attention, notice how she is so present in this moment, feel her love radiating toward you. Absorb it into your heart, and let it flow back again. Let this mutual interaction develop and increase, breathing in love from your baby, breathing out love to your baby.

So calm, so peaceful.

Quietly, softly, focus on the present moment.

Notice the tenderness between you developing in this mutual exchange of love.

Notice how much your baby likes playing this love game with you.

Continue with your deep and focused breathing until your baby has finished feeding.

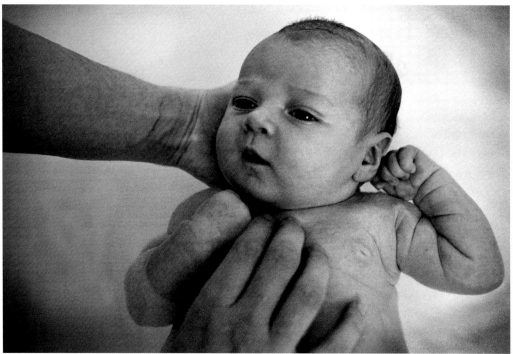

Massage, as an enjoyable activity, helps our babies relax into their bodies.

Touch and massage for babies

Baby massage is really simple. We all know how to do it. There are many courses being run teaching mothers to massage their babies. Some of them are very good. We instinctively know how to touch our babies, though, so all it requires is bringing quiet and focused attention to our touch and setting time aside to simply enjoy soothing our babies through touch.

Infant orphans who are not touched and are not responded to, stop crying once they realize that it is a waste of their energy. Then they withdraw into themselves, seemingly requiring little outside interaction. The numbers of these infants who die without reason is huge compared to infants who receive love and care from birth. Possibly, if they have no contact with human warmth and love, they have no real reason for living.

Studies have shown us that infants who received "massage therapy versus those who were rocked experienced greater daily weight gain, more organized sleep/wake behaviors, less fussiness, improved sociability and soothability, improved interaction behaviors, and lower cortisol and norepinephrine and increased serotonin levels".[112]

Find a warm place to massage your baby—often half an hour after a meal is a good time. It is important to introduce massage when your baby is indicating that this is a time that they welcome your touch. Do this a little bit at a time. In the same way that babies might find bathing a little startling in the first few days, so massage can seem different, perhaps slightly alarming, initially.

Always make sure you are settled and relaxed before starting. Take in a few deep breaths, spending some moments feeling the sensations in your own body, breathing in calm and breathing out tension. Bring your attention to your baby. Smile and chat a bit. Tell him what you'll be doing together. Ask his permission, and don't begin unless you have some reciprocal attention from him, showing you that he is quietly alert.

Apparently, babies respond better to massage with oil than without. Use unscented, cold-pressed vegetable oil rather than processed mineral oil. Warm the oil in your hands first. Use gentle and soft, yet firm strokes—strokes that show your baby that you can support him and keep him safe. Simply holding him quietly with your hands in a "containment" position is often more welcomed initially. Move slowly and surely. Babies love to be sung to with lullabies during a massage—make up your own songs and lyrics if you like. The more often you repeat the same songs, the more wonderful they're likely to sound to him.

Let your baby move around, massaging those areas that he responds to positively. You can use your thumbs on his hands, feet, and ears. Always massage his tummy in a clockwise direction, since that is the direction of his digestive tract, so it will help to move gas and food.

Remember that even though there are all sorts of different massage strokes and routines, this is not a technique; it is an interactive process. The purpose of massaging your baby is to build a warm and loving relationship with him, where he feels secure and has your undivided attention.

Falling apart

Babies are mind-blowingly wonderful. Filled with non-judgmental acceptance, unconditional love, they look like perfect angels when they are sleeping.

What about when they're being bloody awful, though? They scream with colic as babies, scream with frustration as toddlers, scream with anger as teenagers, and then after nursing them through all that and growing them up to be beautiful people, they gently reject you as they leave home and find more interesting lives to lead and people to live among.

As with most problems, the solutions are very simple, albeit sometimes very difficult to enact, and with small variations, are the same for each situation. Since this is a baby book, we'll focus on how to handle falling apart when faced with a with colicky baby.

Most importantly, you need to **look after yourself**. If you're exhausted and bleary eyed and feeling at your wits' end, when your baby hits 6 p.m. and starts screaming, you're not going to be able to maintain any sustainable tranquility that allows you to soothe him out of the pain he is in. Besides, how will you possibly enjoy your baby's early months if you're feeling completely drained and your nerves are on edge?

Sleep whenever you can. Consciously relax. Take some time outside for yourself. Breathe deeply, and simply look around at the world outside of babyhood. Bring your attention into this moment, over and over, and let some of those moments be baby-free ones. If your baby frequently cries as evening approaches, try to rest and take time just for yourself between 4:00 p.m. and 5:00 p.m. It is remarkable the difference this can make to his crankiness.

Once you are feeling a little more centered, **be open** to whatever is happening right now. If your baby loves you, love him back. If he's arching back away from you and moaning, squirming, and screaming, stay open to the feelings you are experiencing as this occurs, probably helplessness, frustration, resentment, or perhaps even despair, usually mixed in with a whole lot of love. It's difficult to do this if you're tired; it's difficult enough when you're not tired. But you will find the more you can surrender into allowing the situation to be just the way it is, the more quickly and easily it will resolve itself.

Babies and mothers have such an integrated energy field in the first few months after birth that babies respond superbly to **relaxation and peacefulness** held in your body if it is really genuine. And it can only be genuine if you always allow the uncomfortable experiences to be as fully present as the wonderful ones.

Don't judge yourself. Many mothers these days have been high-powered executives before their maternal career, and they are used to being perfectly in control, very organized, and capable of managing crises as they arise—smoothly, diplomatically, in a way that allows everyone to remain unruffled. One tiny baby can destroy that image fast. Unless you made enough money as the executive to hire a night nurse, a nanny, and a full-time cleaner, you should be prepared to surrender into the possibility of unwashed hair, unbrushed teeth, unmade beds, and days on end spent doing what seems like nothing at all, but which leaves you harassed and exhausted. If you're not okay with this, you might fall apart simply from the huge dip in self-esteem that can arise from your self-image crumbling to dust.

Don't believe the baby magazines with glowing, perfect earth mothers, or the friends with babies who seem to be coping brilliantly. It's all a show, staged to sell magazines and the friends can't deal with a crushed self-image. Underneath, your friends are likely to be just as exhausted as you are.

Try a joint **cranio-sacral treatment** for yourself and your baby. This soothing, non-invasive touch therapy is related to osteopathy but performed at a light, energetic level. It calms the nervous system and helps the body gently release birth traumas and other problems and feels very relaxing to Mom and baby. Chiropractic help can be equally good, if performed gently. Find any bodywork therapist who can help you and your baby unwind the residual tension from the birth itself. This tension can lock itself into both your bodies, often around the spine, and cause stressed nerves that translate into digestive disorders for your baby and low energy for yourself. Often birth trauma, physical or emotional, can create tension in the digestive tract in young babies. It can be helpful for you both to receive the session since your baby will be reflecting how you are feeling as well, particularly if the birth was stressful for both of you. I recommend that all mother and babies should have a cranio-sacral session within the first few weeks after birth. For colicky pain and crying, you can try pressing the base of the spine *very gently* on the sacrum and the lower lumbar vertebrae. There is a point there which helps to release gas. A baby needs only the very gentlest pressure, no more than a gentle rub. Drawing your fingers gently down on either side of the spine can help, too.

Meditation prior to and during breast-feeding can help to slow you down into present-moment awareness. Its purpose is to help you relax and unwind prior to the tension exploding build-up that may occur for your baby at certain times of day. We all hold onto beliefs about pregnancy, birth, and parenting. Beliefs such as I should be glowing and happy because I'm pregnant, so why am I feeling sick and miserable? Or childbirth is the most painful experience you'll ever encounter. Or babies should sleep through by three months. Meditation helps us to recognize that these beliefs are simply other people's ideas of how things should be, which impact on our actual experience of how things really are.

Responding to baby signals

Often having birthed our first babies, we find ourselves, less than twenty-four hours later, in a situation where as new parents we are expected to take care of them, on our own, with *no idea* or previous experience of how to manage them or interpret their signals. Then within a week they are showing us how truly inadequate and inexperienced we really feel by tensing up with colic and reflux and inconsolable crying.

There are many reasons for colic: physical trauma from the birth can often cause colic, and chiropractic or craniosacral work can be enormously helpful in relieving symptoms of colic in newborns.

In the event of being unable to find other reasons for your baby's distress, it might be worthwhile noticing if they are picking up on any stress that you may be carrying. Since babies are so sensitive to our feelings, it is possible for them to pick up on any unease and hold it physically in their bodies. It can require great courage to stay with the uncomfortable feelings in situations created by colicky babies (or frustrated two-year-olds, or angry teenagers) when our natural inclination is to resist them and react by getting tense and distressed ourselves. Especially if we find that when we do open up and simply allow the feelings to be there, they might not go away immediately; we may be required to open to them on a deeper level still.

Feeling some resentment mixed with anxiety toward a screaming baby who simply won't be comforted is one level of opening. Moving deeper into that feeling can expose what lies beneath, which may be great resistance to the sensations of having once been in a similar situation as a baby ourselves. Those memories, which are stored in our precognitive minds, may include feelings of being out of control, or perhaps feelings of bewilderment at being in this constricting body that is causing such pain and fear. We may have experienced these sensations because of our own mother's anxiety, causing us to intuit that we couldn't truly trust the world in which we lived, because perhaps she didn't either.

It is a lot to expect of our own babies that they should let go of these patterns and be easily comforted when we are holding onto similar memories ourselves. If our baby is to feel truly at home in this world, then we must feel okay in ourselves, too. To feel deeply okay we need to allow that it was truly alright for us to have experienced similar discomfort.

Sometimes the most comforting thing for a baby is to allow her to cry, while simply holding her, without needing her to stop, allowing the feelings that arise from listening to her crying, to simply reveal themselves to you, just allowing yourself to truly feel them, no matter how uncomfortable. The relief she can experience from your ability to be honest with your body and the sensations being held there can be enormous.

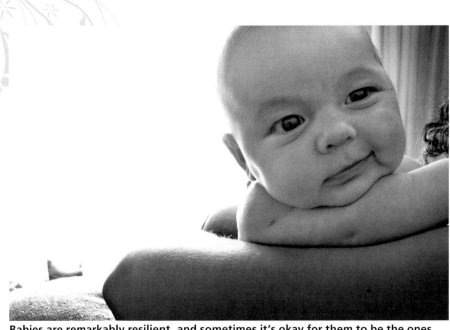

Babies are remarkably resilient, and sometimes it's okay for them to be the ones supporting us with their smiles and their humor.

How we respond to the experiences we encounter impacts those around us. So when we encounter a loved baby in pain, causing us to feel pain ourselves, we are responsible for staying open enough to our experience to be able to resolve it for ourselves. In doing so, we can break the pattern for our baby—or child, or teenager.

Breaking patterns that have been entrenched for generations is difficult, but it is awesome work. It teaches us to love ourselves just the way we are, and to develop enormous empathy for those around us, even for the people who taught us those patterns in the first place, because they didn't know any better themselves.

Jan runs Comacare at Groote Schuur Hospital in Cape Town. Comacare is like a hospice for people in a coma. Most of Jan's "teachers"—other people would call them patients—are between the ages of sixteen and twenty-five and are in a coma as a result of drug and alcohol abuse, driving accidents, or violent behavior. Sometimes, the staff members at the hospital think the patients deserve their fate, given their past lifestyles. Except Jan. Jan listens to her teachers without any judgment. She listens by observing finger twitches, eye movements, grunts and grimaces, expressions of peacefulness or anguish. All of it is just okay to Jan. She listens and reflects back to them, so that on some level they know that they are heard and that somebody cares.

I want to package Jan up and take her home from the talk she's giving about her work, so that she can listen to me like that. Then when she's finished doing that, I want her to teach all the parents I work with how to listen to their babies. Perhaps, as parents, we should all go on Comacare courses.

Babies, like coma patients, are hypersensitive to the emotional atmosphere surrounding them, and like coma patients, they are seldom able to do a lot about it. They can only cry, which is counterproductive, since it's likely to make the atmosphere even more tense, or learn to smile really fast, which can be difficult after the shock of birth.

Getting to know our babies, particularly when we don't understand their language yet, requires Jan-like attention. Babies thrive on that kind of love. They grow better and fatter and happier under our gaze. Slowing down our breathing, taking time, noticing their soft bellies and milky breath makes them content. Perhaps it's a baby's job to teach us that kind of awareness, and then they can simply settle in to the feeling of a job well done when we really listen to them.

Finally, the most important part of any of these exercises is to recognize that sometimes, babies just cry. Sometimes, they have a hard time fitting into their little bodies. Sometimes all the self-awareness and noble relaxation on their behalf just isn't going to crack it for them. Sometimes, all we can do is love them through those early months. Being perfect just isn't what it's all about.

Crying meditation

Try this meditation during a colicky episode with your baby. Read it through beforehand and improvize like crazy. It is important not to place an extra burden of guilt and blame on yourself if you feel that your baby might be picking up on your own suppressed grief or fear. This is simply an extra tool for managing colicky episodes if other avenues may have failed thus far.

If you can manage to do so, try to get a little centered and present before any crying starts. This may be helpful simply because our deepest grief can be so well concealed that it may be difficult to access if we are not fully present and aware of how we are really feeling. This is precisely why it is such a gift from our babies to be given a doorway into that grief in order to be helped to release it.

When your baby starts crying with colic, simply allow her to do so without trying to pacify or shush her. Hold her and love her, but don't try to quieten her. Often babies >

need to cry out some residual tension from their birth. As a parent, this is a difficult exercise. Instinctively we want to rescue our baby from the pain they are experiencing. Instead, try to see what her crying does to you. How does it make you feel? In your heart? In your chest? In your solar plexus? In your stomach? Describe the sensations to yourself. Then ask yourself some of the following questions, and feel deeply in your body for the answers: Is your baby crying for you, because you've forgotten how to cry yourself? Do you still remember how to cry like a baby? Did you cry as much as you needed to when you were one month old, or did your mother perhaps try desperately to shush you because it was too painful for her to stay open to your crying?

Did you cry as a baby because you felt the suppressed pain that your parents were holding—crying for your own mother and for the grief she was never allowed to feel herself? Is this yet another pattern of resistance that plays out through the Red Thread of descendancy and through generations of deeply held grief and sadness? Do you feel overwhelmed right now? Too grown up? Do you feel like you'll never be the old, fun-filled you again?

Allow yourself to feel sad for the parts of you that are uncomfortable. Are there places in your body that are feeling as if they really can't cope with your baby crying? Often, if we can feel enough empathy for ourselves that we allow ourselves to cry, it can be an enormous relief for our babies. They often fall asleep when we start to feel our own pain, as if they acknowledge the relief of no longer having to carry our feelings for us, because we are now responsible enough to hold those feelings for ourselves.

Try then to simply stay present with any negative feelings that are resonating in your own body. Try to cry for yourself, caught in this web of adult-like expectations amid the chaos of holding onto a struggling, squirming baby who quite simply won't be soothed. How does it really feel? Because it's a helluva job, and it's completely okay to feel sorry for yourself. Acknowledging your own needs is as important for the babies being born these days as taking care of theirs.

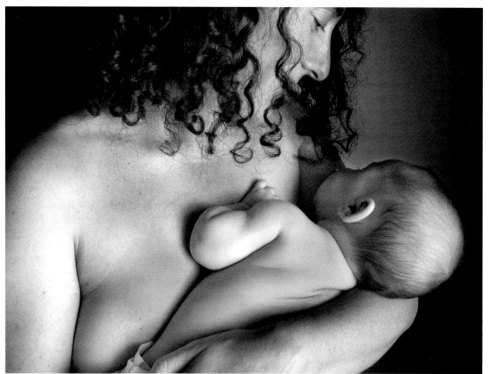

If we can feel our own pain, exhaustion, or fear about parenting, then our babies don't have to energetically hold it for us. Looking after yourself is the first step to helping your baby enjoy life.

A new mother mentioned that she felt as if she had given up forever her old life, which was sometimes fun and frivolous. She felt that ultimately nobody else could fix this situation for her, so she resented the fact that her husband and her relations tried to help with advice and worrying, because it truly seemed like she was entirely responsible for her baby's happiness, and that even her husband was not able to help very much.

A midwife, who had two babies who were both colicky and who is a tremendous support to mothers in similar situations, said that having her babies was the time in her life when she first learned how not to cry. Suddenly there was the expectation of having to hold it all together and be the grownup. No longer were things simply allowed to unravel, and that part of her that couldn't cope desperately longed for someone else to hold her, rock her, and soothe her, crooning, "there there, it's all going to be okay now, I'm here to look after you."

This feeling of being overwhelmed might be raw and easy for your newborn to connect to. You might be too tired to care about your needs. Taking care of a crying baby is emotionally stressful as it is; to have to also work on staying open to your own stress and despair might be more than you feel ready to cope with.

However, mourning your own losses can help you release your own frustration, despair, and grief. It may suddenly make the sun come out. Having a good cry yourself might just change the whole situation around and bring relief to you all. It truly can't do any harm to try.

Pre-verbal communication

According to Credo Mutwa, a Zulu shaman and author of *Indaba My Children*, in African folklore it is believed that man used to live in a type of paradise, much like the Garden of Eden. In those days everyone communicated with the power of the mind, or mental telepathy. The fall of man occurred when he was given the power of speech. This power divided men, and they could no longer properly understand or communicate with one another. Ever since then there have been quarrels and wars on Earth.

It is remarkably easy to communicate with babies using mental imagery. Being preverbal, it is easier to imagine their "messages" and for them to pick up your mental images than it is once your child has learned to communicate with words. Firstborn children usually learn to talk earlier than their siblings because their parents are not communicating much with them on a preverbal level. When a sibling arrives, the firstborn child can still remember preverbal communication and easily understand their younger siblings' needs. Therefore , second- and third-born children don't bother to learn language as quickly because they can communicate through their older brother or sister, who translates their communications into language for them.

It is easiest to establish communication through mental imagery when our babies are contented initially. We can communicate with them by slowing down to their pace, breathing quietly, bringing awareness to our bodies, and settling into the present moment. Thereafter, with eyes closed or open, just imagine what your child is feeling. Ask specific questions, like "How are you feeling?" or "What do you think of this new room?" Write your answers down immediately you imagine them. You may receive an image. You may hear your own voice in your head seemingly making it all up. You may get a feeling, for instance, of peacefulness or discomfort if you ask "How are you feeling?" It is remarkably easy and

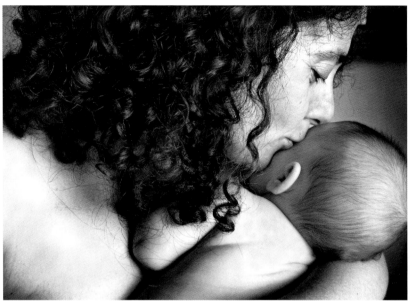

Preverbal communication happens through mental imagery, through signals like kissing, and through feelings like love.

you only learn to trust this type of communication through writing it down and through repetition. If we watch our babies' responses to how they like being communicated with in this way, it will also give us confidence in the method.

Yesterday, I was working with two women with two- and four-month-old babies, one awake, the other asleep. As the women silently asked the question of their babies, "How are you doing?" both babies immediately smiled broadly and visibly settled in their bodies.

Baby-naming ceremony

Blessing a newborn and giving your baby her name is a sacred act. It is wonderful to acknowledge your baby with a ceremony in her honor.

Be consciously aware of your choice of name for your baby and allow the name to express your child's personality or how you feel about them. Even if the name has come to you in a dream or from a sibling's insistence that this is the correct name, find out the meaning of the name; usually, it will communicate something you had intuitively or openly felt about the child anyway.

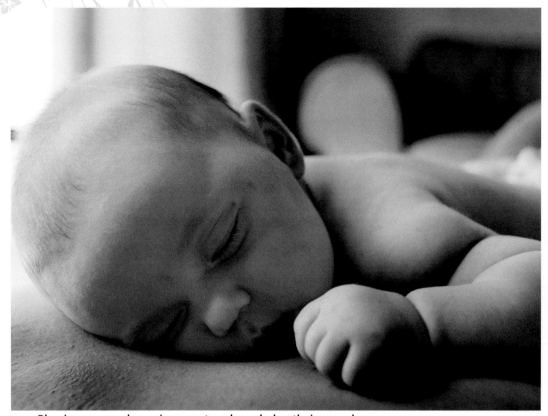

Blessing our newborns is a way to acknowledge their sacredness.

Often parents choose a child's name simply because it feels good to them and often these names will describe how they feel about the child. My own children were named way back before I was aware that the meaning of names might be significant, and yet each of them has a name that suits their personality.

Consider where and when you might want to hold the ceremony. Often, parents choose to hold the ceremony outdoors, perhaps on a full moon or in a place that feels sacred or special. The intention with which we create rituals is as important as the ritual itself, so consider each aspect of the ritual with care. Plan the ceremony with the awareness that each detail of the ceremony has symbolic significance. Give as much consideration to the colors, clothing, flowers, venue, and timing as you do to the wording of the ceremony itself.

Use ideas that have meaning for you at the ceremony, and draw them from various traditions if you feel attracted to them.

Usually a baby-naming ceremony consists of all or some of the following elements:
- Welcoming the baby into the community.
- Announcing the names of the child.
- Blessing the child and making commitments. This is the opportunity for family members and friends to be 'honored' by their inclusion in the ceremony, by the reading of a poem or special verse, by offering prayers for the child (this can be very important for grandparents whose children have no particular religious adherence), singing, etcetera. Often, the child wears a special gown that may have a long family tradition, or be made from the mother's wedding dress, or be otherwise specially made for the purpose, and thus commence a family tradition.
- Choosing guardians/godparents/spiritual caregivers for the child.

66 Vulnerable we are, like an infant.
We need each other's care
Or we will
Suffer. 99
— *St. Catherine of Siena, Patron Saint of Italy, 1347–1380* [113]

LOSS OF A BABY

Chapter Seven

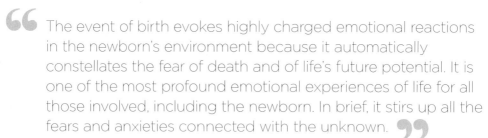

" The event of birth evokes highly charged emotional reactions in the newborn's environment because it automatically constellates the fear of death and of life's future potential. It is one of the most profound emotional experiences of life for all those involved, including the newborn. In brief, it stirs up all the fears and anxieties connected with the unknown. "

— *Mara Sidoli, Jungian analyst* [114]

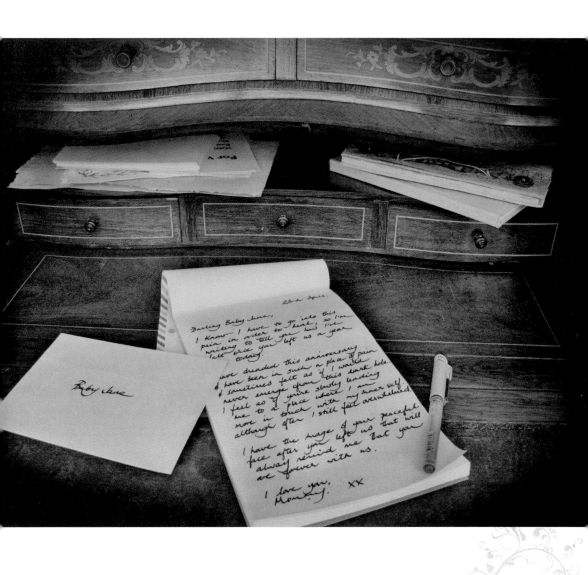

Death and grief

> Then a woman said, Speak to us of Joy and Sorrow.
> And he answered:
> Your joy is your sorrow unmasked.
> And the self-same well from which your laughter rises
> was oftentimes filled with your tears.
>
> — *Kahlil Gibran, Poet, philosopher, theologian, 1883–1931* [115]

Death doesn't seem to have a place in a book on birth. Yet, for those who face it, it belongs here and will not easily be denied. Trusting birth, letting go into the process of birth does not require that we trust birth's outcome. We do not know where life and our babies will lead us. Trust is simply a progression of staying with what is and of trusting our ability to respond authentically to each moment. Trust is a method of feeling our way through life, rather like a blind man who does not know what is ahead of him, and who can allow that that, too, is okay.

This seems a simple enough task if we're feeling loved and happy, but can be frustrating when we're stuck in front of long-ignored cash-flow balances, or heart-rending when loved ones are in pain or suffering. Way beyond this concept of trusting life lays the concept of how we react in the face of having someone we love die.

Death is shocking. It tears us apart and leaves us raw and wounded. The indivisible connection between life and death is clearly felt at birth. New life entering this world feels fragile, not because newborns die easily—they are remarkably resilient—but because the baby is still hovering on the brink between fully entering life and leaving behind a more cosmic consciousness. The time of birth has a shocking tenderness to it that is often similar to the atmosphere surrounding a person leaving their body.

Yet even though there is this strange connection between new life and death, when a baby dies it always feels wrong. To not even have a real chance at life is not fair, and doesn't fit into the proper order where the old people are supposed to die before the young ones. The loss of a baby is devastating, whether it is before birth, at birth, or in infancy. The idea of loving life enough to include even death, especially in the context of a baby, seems callous and ridiculously hurtful.

How can anyone rightfully love death? The idea is an oxymoron, a terrible marrying of opposites. However, beneath the awfulness of losing a loved one, deep beneath our desire to be anywhere other than in such a place of grief, beneath the experience of being overwhelmed and washed through by our despair, or worse, numb to our core, lies the experience of life itself. The surrender at odd moments into life's encounters is not a passive giving up, but rather a movement toward undiscriminating love, which embraces all that life has to offer.

When we are in mourning, we can experience moments of clarity that are not revealed by mundane existence. Author and spiritual teacher, Andrew Harvey, is a man who has learned to embrace all of life extravagantly, despite its difficulties. In an interview in *The Eight Faces of Eve*, he describes the enjoyment of recognizing miracles in everyday existence. Then he adds "And the difficulty is to see Her [the Divine Mother's] presence in pain and suffering and death and darkness. But that comes later, through an initiation into heartbreak, and the acceptance of the price of love."[116]

Hearts can become very soft at times of grief because the barriers we put up to protect ourselves from the world have all been smashed. Feelings at the time of a baby's death can be utterly overwhelming, and loving in this context can only mean surrendering to the process of grief, moment by moment, over and over, for days, weeks, months, years. The loss of a baby also involves the loss of all the dreams and fantasies about the baby, extending far into the future. The contrast of birth and death, when occurring simultaneously without the expected lifetime in-between may seem incomprehensible to parents, and the healthy expression of grief is an important part of the process of recovery. Grief may also occur to a lesser degree over smaller losses during the childbirth period, such as loss of independence, loss of the closeness felt with the fetus in the womb, or loss of expectations for a perfect baby and a perfect birth.

The loss of a child changes our lives as parents forever. Losing a baby is not something we get over soon, if ever. A new pregnancy or medication will not help us forget the loss; we won't forget—we are not meant to forget. Grieving for a long time isn't a sign of an inability to cope. Some days and some months will be worse than others. Parents may feel they have come to terms with the death, only to have a new wave of grief hit them a month later.

In the First World, sometimes the loss of an infant is the parent's first encounter with grief. Bertha Simos writes in *A Time to Grieve* that, "It is a mistake to think that time alone will heal the pain of grief. It is how time is used that will be a factor in determining how long the pain remains acute, whether it is even fully experienced, and how long it will take for recovery.... The feeling must be accurately perceived, experienced, identified by its right name (for example, shame and guilt are not the same), endured, and finally mastered through sufficient expression and discharge.... Grief is an active, not a passive process; Freud rightfully labeled it "work." It is mental and emotional labor. It is exhaustive and exhausting, not only for the bereaved but also for those about them and those who would be of comfort to them."[117]

It is important to recognize that grief is normal, and the work of moving through the stages of grief is essential for keeping grief normal. Suppression of the emotions associated with grief, and a refusal to work through these emotions, can lead to a morbid, pathological grief reaction. We need to be aware that the ability to grieve is also the ability to enjoy life—suppression of grief must also decrease the space we have in our bodies for enjoyment or for any other emotions.

Culturally, we have been taught to avoid the grief process: we try to protect our children from funerals, we cover the raw earth at the graveside with a green carpet, we have funeral directors take the body away, and if we see it at all, it has been made up to look as "nice" as possible. We live, in fact, in a grief-denying culture. Older traditions honor the process of grieving, and mourners are often required to express their feelings at funerals. In the Jewish tradition, "Kriyah," or the rending of garments at a funeral, symbolizes the internal tearing asunder that the mourner feels in his relationship with the deceased.

However, there is no way to "grieve correctly." There is just being with what is as whole-heartedly as the moment allows. The feeling of not grieving correctly, of being separate, even from our grief, is the work of grieving. Grief is not new to us; grief at the loss of a baby is the intensification of emotions that we already know, and usually manage to avoid feeling. However, when the loss is so enormous, it becomes almost impossible to avoid any longer. Meditation teacher and hospice worker Stephen Levine says that, "It is that fact of separation from ourselves and others, which most accurately describes grief… When we begin to acknowledge our everyday sense of isolation from that which we love most and wish so dearly to merge with, we begin to let go of the grief and pain which has always existed around our hearts."[118] We cannot let go of anything we do not accept, so the work of grief is to slowly open up to those emotions, which most of us would prefer to run away from.

> What we find when we listen to the songs of our rage or fear, loneliness or longing, is that they do not stay forever. Rage turns into sorrow; sorrow turns into tears; tears may fall for a long time, but then the sun comes out… loss sings to us; our body shakes and relives the moment of loss; then the armoring around that loss gradually softens; and in the midst of the song of tremendous grieving, the pain of that loss finally finds release.

— *Jack Kornfield, Buddhist teacher, and psychotherapist* [119]

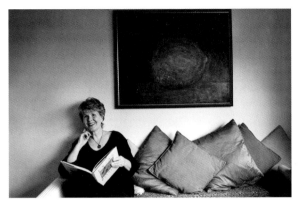

Andrée.

Andrée and Adam's story

A couple of months ago, my teenage daughter, Lisa, unexpectedly turned to me and said: "I'm going to call my son Adam." I was surprised. We don't talk about him much. After all, he died in my arms eighteen years ago, two years before she was born.

Her statement provoked memories. Once again. And for a few days I was plunged headlong into yet another stint of grief. Shortly afterwards, I was invited to share Adam's story as a contribution to this book.

In keeping with the way synchronicity operates, I was unable to meet with Robyn at the time. It was December, and I was preparing for a holiday away from home, so we moved our meeting back to January. At the beginning of January I was returning home after my holiday, and on the flight, a few rows ahead of me, sat a tall, blond young man who captivated my attention. I could not take my eyes off him. I stared at his lean, sun-tanned physique. This, I thought, is what Adam would have looked like. He was with some friends, and I marveled at his playfulness, his exuberance, as he interacted with them. I was projecting all my hopeless dreams on this boy, and for a few brief minutes my fantasy sustained me, until the cold hand of fact ripped the fragile dream to pieces and I was left sitting in an uncomfortable plane seat to deal with the after-effects. That sinking in the pit of the stomach. That sickening disappointment. He's gone, he's been gone for eighteen years, for God's sake, get real!

A few days later—still in January—I had a dream about a baby dying in my arms, and I woke up crying tears that were more salty than usual, as old, dormant tears are. I lay in bed, drenched not only with tears but also with a sharp, piercing yearning for a >

child I never knew, and I was swept into a lucid memory of the events that surrounded his death. Blow by blow, I experienced once again the full impact of his death, as if it were happening in the present.

By the time dawn stole into my room, I had managed to surface from revisiting the past. I reflected on how, just when I had imagined that I was healed of the torment of grief, Lisa's casual remark had pushed it all to the surface again and had given rise to a series of experiences that related to Adam. It was then that I realized that these experiences all occurred in January, and it was in the month of January that Adam died!

I was reminded again that the cells of grief lie dormant and can be triggered at the most unexpected times. And how mysterious it is that every January, even when I am fully occupied with the demands of life, a hidden, automatic, memory-button gets pushed which reactivates the past.

As I sat up in bed, thinking about the intense whirlwind of "January grief" that visited me again, I reflected on how I had developed resources to deal with the pain over the years. That way, when grief strikes, it at least does not linger over an extended period, and it does not become a constant, crippling pain.

By mid-morning, the night's raw sorrow—which defied all attempts at self-comfort and made every perspective on grief appear glib and mere lip service—could be transmuted into tender sadness. Like one season melts into another, this poignancy turned, by mid-afternoon, to a deep and tender sense of the human condition. No one is spared grief, in one form or another. By the end of the day I thought of how all loss is ultimately an opportunity to refine the art of being a messenger of love, and how this is the only attitude that, for me, makes any sense at all of destiny's brutal demands.

It was 1989. My husband, Johann, and I waited for our son with ardent enthusiasm. Our daughter, Leandra, who was four, shared our anticipation in her childlike way. Johann and I were halfway through a writing project at the time of my pregnancy, and I felt compelled to complete it before the baby arrived. I worked tirelessly. At twenty-seven weeks, while driving with Johann to conduct an interview for our book, I went into labor.

The gynecologist on duty in the local hospital stood by my bed shortly after my waters broke. I was shaking, out of control, terrified. I pleaded for consolation: "Am I going to lose this child? Can't you stop this from happening?" He looked down at me, and *asked, notably irritated, why I was shaking. While I was assaulted by the pains of a labor of which I knew the horrible outcome, he suggested that I pull myself together.*

I was wheeled to a theatre. Johann walked by my side. Within minutes my child slipped from my body. I heard a plaintive cry. It sounded like a desperate, exhausted, little animal, but it was my son. He was taken from me, in great haste, to be examined. Johann followed, and I was returned to the ward.

A drip was inserted into my arm. All was unreal. Johann returned with a pediatrician, who informed me that our baby was underdeveloped; he had no reflexes, and he would die within hours. The doctor assured us that instead of mourning a loss, we should regard this unfortunate turn of events as a blessing. We were being released from the lifetime of suffering that a brain-damaged child would bring.

A nurse brought my child to me, and Johann, looking dazed, left for home to tell Leandra that the brother she was waiting for would not live. I was alone with a beautiful, perfectly formed baby boy in my arms.

I turned back the blanket in which he was wrapped to look at him. I stroked his soft skin. I noticed that he looked just like Leandra did when she was born. I whispered, "Adam, I love you." I prayed. I offered him up to God. I invoked every possible assistance for an easy, pain-free release. I held him close. I gazed at him with adoration. He did not seem to be in pain. His tiny puffs of breath gradually became weaker. After an hour, Adam died in my arms.

A nurse came in and took him from me. In view of the fact, she said, that premature babies are not considered to be "legal," they don't count as human beings, so there are no formalities to be considered. Adam would be incinerated by the hospital. I listened and complied. I wondered why I felt so calm. I lay back in bed. The drip was still half-full.

My mother, my sister, and my sister-in-law came to fetch me. They were tender, but not one of them seemed to be available to me, emotionally. It felt as if I had crossed into a world where I was chillingly alone. So I numbed my feelings, and I rationalized my grief. My baby was not real. He would have been abnormal, had he survived, so the best I could do was to go home and get on with life.

Back home, my family urged me to fall pregnant as soon as I could. My husband repeated the words of the pediatrician. It all made perfect sense.

The next day, everything changed. Numb compliance became bottomless grief. I found myself lying on my stomach in our darkened bedroom. My breasts were engorged with milk. I swam for my life in a tempest of tears. No one was available to give >

me a hand. I thought I would drown. There was no land in sight. I could find no way out by myself, and so, once again, I buried my pain.

My trauma in that dark room was dominated by two themes, which caused acute mental suffering for years. I will deal with them one at a time.

Firstly, I was shocked that I had given up the body of my child to the indifference of nursing staff. How could I, a woman who feels deeply, a mother who loves deeply, how could I comply with rules that totally ignored the human experience? How could I not have insisted on some closing ceremony shared with Johann and Leandra?

With the wisdom of hindsight, I have a clearer understanding of why I acted in that way. Very possibly, I was heavily sedated by what was in the drip. And, of course, I was numbed by shock. But most of all, I lacked confidence in my own authentic responses. I was never taught to be fiercely proud of being a woman, and of valuing the heartfelt response which is the natural way of a woman's being.

A dismissive gynecologist who reprimanded me for displaying symptoms of shock, quickly convinced me to shut up. A nurse who informed me that Adam was not "human" and, therefore, his little body would be disposed of so clinically, was left unchallenged. My family's attitude that we should move on (even if they acted in a spirit of love, and this was their way to make me feel better) left me mute. My husband tried to comfort me by urging me to look ahead. But I needed to mourn the past. The problem was that I could not find the words to explain this to him.

Had I, lying on that white, starched bed with a dead baby in my arms, only been shamelessly connected to my primal female nature, I would have known that giving over to the immense grief of a bereft mother, despite what anyone else believed, would facilitate my healing. I would have wrapped that little body in a soft blanket and appealed to Johann to join with me, and Leandra, in marking the end of a cycle.

Had I honored myself more, I would have known that life's deepest losses cannot be carried in stoic solitude. I would have sought appropriate help and guidance through the quagmire of grief. I would have expressed my feelings and known that it is safe to do so. I would have expressed my needs, and known that I am worthy of doing so. I would have been kind to myself and known that it is healthy to do so.

The other theme of those years of slow, persistent self-torture was a morbid sense of guilt. "My single-minded focus to complete a book caused his death," I reprimanded myself. "I exhausted myself. I did not take heed of my body's needs."

I took this belief on and crucified myself on it daily. And as if self-flagellation was not enough, more proof of my culpability was soon to follow.

My mother visited one afternoon. We discussed again the sequence of events that led to Adam's death. Why did I go into labor? Was the doctor in whose care I was negligent? I was struggling to make sense of my grief and hoped for a motherly touch, a supportive word. Instead, out of the blue, she remarked, "You should have been more careful." In that moment, every confidence I had about my ability to mother Leandra, every instinctual connection I had ever had to myself as a mother, shattered.

Shortly after this, I consulted a medium. I needed answers to the maddening turmoil in my mind. I sat in front of a woman who, I hoped, would provide me with the comfort of a higher perspective. But to my horror, she said with alarm in her voice: "But this should not have happened!" Seconds later, she corrected herself and commented that, in fact, it was Adam's choice to go so soon. But the message I resonated with was already drummed into my brain: I was guilty of the worst crime possible. By not being vigilant, by trying to get work done, by not being a good mother, I had somehow allowed this horrible fate to unfold. The will of God had been twisted by my own negligence.

It took years to un-crucify myself.

Learning to forgive myself for my belief that I caused Adam's death was a long process that was not chronological or well-defined and did not come in a neatly packaged series of processes. It was fluid and often confusing and punctuated by despair, as much as it was exhilarating and awesome, and it offered peak moments of joy.

I visited therapists, learned releasing techniques, and sought out body-work therapies that assisted the release of pain. But primarily, I was continually reminded that a healthy relationship with myself was the core around which healing revolved. I committed myself to a journey of learning how to become comfortable with myself, and like everyone who chooses this route, I was amazed at the elegance of timing. The right people and tools presented themselves always at the right time.

The path of psychological work (which is ongoing, naturally) bore excellent fruit, and my torment of guilt became manageable. I came to understand so much, even my mother's inept expression of her own fear.

But eventually I stumbled upon another path, also—a much more obscure path, without much foothold. It is a path on which all signposts are maddeningly conflicting, and nothing makes sense, and I am forced, minute by minute, to call out, "I don't >

understand!" Strangely, on this path, the more I give up trying to understand, the more I realize that my habit of self-attack is an attempt at controling life. The most gracious thing, for myself and for those around me, is to stand aside and let life happen. Despite every opinion, no one knows why some babies die and some live. How do I know that Adam was meant to die? Because he did.

Life is a mystery, and there is great peace in saying yes to the unfolding of destiny, which surges along, despite my best efforts to channel it into a direction that suits my plans. As my spiritual teacher says, when asked about death, "Coming in and going out is the Lord's domain."

I now accept that my human needs sometimes defy all the wisdom that I may have gathered. There are—and there will almost certainly always be—times when nothing, no resource, no well-meaning friend, no spiritual tool, can stop the tears, and all comfort appears facile in the face of the yearning to see my son again.

Yet the greatest peace, which defies all logic, comes when I am able to bow to the wisdom of a Greater Will, and to open my hands to the way things are.

Having received this beautiful account from Andrée Eva Bosch via e-mail, we decided we still wanted to meet to talk about her experiences and see what came up in our discussion. We spoke about all her births, about life, about being honest with ourselves in the face of our experiences, and in a quiet moment when we were simply sitting with what else needed to be said, she received an impression that Adam clearly needed to be heard. We sat quietly for a while more for her to intuit the things she felt he wanted to say. The wisdom that she and Adam passed on for all women who have lost children was painful for her to express. Eighteen years after his death, listening to her speaking, it felt as though this pain at losing a child, which is carried like a scar, brings with it extraordinary empathy, insight, and compassion:

Adam is often in my presence, like now. A gentle breeze, he visits me. And when I listen closely, he tells me that I would be free from the weight of grief if I remember that the soul is eternal and that our connection is never severed. It remains a relationship, and it is as worthy of celebration as any other.

He helps me understand, in intimate moments like these, that a particularly strong grace is bestowed on every parent who has lost a child… and an image comes up of us, a collective group of parents, who are all held very close to the Great Comforter.

Because no other loss defies the natural order of things as savagely as this one, and no other loss reaches as deep, we who have watched them slip away are left with hearts broken open.

So, Adam whispers, instead of regarding ourselves only as bereft, we should regard ourselves also as recipients. Recipients of open hearts. And open hearts can hold, and give, not trickles, but torrents of love.

Stages in the grieving process

When a child dies, our secure sense of where we are placed in life, that sense of solidity which we rely on to negotiate our way through every day can dissolve into either a blurry haze or a frightening clarity, neither of which have clear boundaries for relating to the world. At times like this, a description of what to expect from the grieving process may provide a sense of some structure for the months ahead.

Grief manifests in many guises. It is a generic label for a specific process that can include agitation, anger, anxiety, feeling lost, guilt, shame, self-doubting, and so on. Parents often expect to feel sad, but may be unprepared for some of the other emotions that can be overwhelming at this time. *Varney's Midwifery Manual* [120] describes three stages of grief as shock, suffering, and resolution. In fact, the emotions of grief often play back and forth between the stages before settling into a final resolution. Each stage of grief has different manifestations, which evolve as we work through the preceding ones. We may not experience all of them, but each phase that arises must be experienced to a peak of intensity before it can be resolved.

According to *Varney's* these stages can be broken down into:

Shock

Denial and isolation

"No, not our baby!" Initial feelings are often of shock and numbness. These feelings may be most intense at the time of the event, but there may be secondary peaks again at two months and at twelve months.

Rage and anger

"Why did this have to happen to us?" This stage can take the form of resentment at the fact that others are healthy and well, while we are bereft and lonely. This may even take the form of feeling anger toward people who have live babies. Elizabeth Kubler Ross refers to God as being a special target for anger, since He is regarded as imposing the death sentence arbitrarily.

Blame

Resentment and blame may focus on God or on a particular person, like the obstetrician or midwife. It may also be aimed at ourselves or our partners, both of which can lead to feelings of shame and guilt.

Bargaining

Often at this stage, we might bargain with God, even if we have never spoken to God before. This stage is particularly significant if our baby hasn't died yet, but is very likely to— for example, if we birth a baby with severe congenital abnormalities.

Suffering

Great overwhelming sadness can arise as the reality of the situation seeps in. During this time, there is likely to be a preoccupation with and idealization of the lost one who died. Events leading to and surrounding our loss are replayed over and over. Feelings of anger, guilt, and fear are still being played out. Questions of "why" and "what if" can become repetitive.

The pain of suffering often comes in "waves," momentarily overwhelming us. Crying is usually a helpful form of release from the totality of this pain. Other emotions we may feel may include vulnerability, anxiety, rage, guilt, apathy, and feelings of loss of control. Emptiness and hopelessness are not signs of a pathological grief reaction; they may be a very real part of the process of releasing the grief.

As parents who have lost a child, we may be told that we should be over it by now; but "getting over it" is not something to be "done," it works its way through us in its own time. As we continue to feel the grief, our preoccupation with our loss gradually changes to reawakening, to awareness that we have a future, albeit a future without our child. This awareness may also lead to anxieties about experiencing loss again.

Many of the emotions that arise hand in hand with grief may not feel appropriate. If we are angry at our baby who died, for any number of reasons, we may not be willing to express it since it may seem dishonorable to them. Working through these ambivalent feelings is necessary to be able to access the sorrow beneath them.

Remember, too, that our hormone production at childbirth, and in the early period after birth, should be helping us to bond more closely, breast-feed more effectively, and, according to Michel Odent, in the case of oxytocin, should be creating intense feelings of love for our babies. It is quite possible, therefore, that these hormones may serve to increase our perceptions of loss at this time.

Resolution and Acceptance

This phase arises with the establishment of new significant relationships. Adjustment is completed, and we once again become fully functional. This stage may take up to a full year to reach, or even longer. Grief at the loss of a baby is never likely to disappear entirely, but over time, given a supportive environment, will usually soften to a more open acceptance of the occurrence—often bringing with it a deeper empathy for others in similar situations.

Pathological grief reactions

The reactions below may occur in the grief process if we are not given the tools to work through the emotions of grief. They do not mean that we are so inadequate that we can't even grieve correctly, but they are a sign that assistance with grieving, usually from a professional, would be helpful.

- **Long-term depression:** This can feel like a gray, hopeless place that we can feel stuck in forever. Suicidal thoughts arise at times.
- **Psychosomatic conditions:** Since most illness is stress related, psychosomatic problems can manifest as severe illnesses at times. There is a very high correlation between cancer and bereavement or loss in the two-year period prior to onset of the cancer.
- **Participating in activities that are detrimental to our social or economic existence,** for example alcohol or drug abuse, to hide from the pain of our loss.
- **An inability to behave in acceptable social patterns of behavior and interaction**
- **Developing a morbid attachment to possessions of our lost baby.**
- **Suffering from a persistent loss of self-esteem.**

How grief can be assisted

Grieving can be assisted by:
- Honest, factual information.
- An acknowledgment of the event.
- Being given choices and options, if at all possible.
- Support, especially from our partners, but also from caregivers, family, friends
- Guidance.
- Comfort—being touched and held by others—empathy and understanding.
- Help in coping with our feelings.
- Help with household chores/financial responsibilities.
- We should be allowed to ask for help, when we feel the need for it. Allowing others to share our pain can be comforting, and friends and family will also feel less helpless.
- Advice—only if and when we ask for it.
- Being able to see and hold our babies after death.
- Gradually developing a realistic perception of the event to allow the loss to become real.
- Relearning how to live without fear and anxiety.
- Reassurance of our sanity, when this is appropriate.
- Recognition of our ability to carry a child, however briefly.
- Developing an ability to trust again that it's okay to love so deeply.
- Support groups/bereavement counseling services.

The period following a death

We need to be listened to and to be looked after in the period following a child's death. Once a day for a month may not be too often.

Except for cremation or burial, we as a culture have few rituals to contain the grief that arises from a death. Often the taboo surrounding death leaves little outlet for these emotions. Parents could write their baby a letter. Let the first things that come to mind be written down, and deeper thoughts will surface. We can tell our babies how we feel, and what has happened to family life since they died. The planting of a tree in honor of our babies is a ritual that can help to acknowledge the loss.

It's okay for us to take as long as we need to grieve. There is no set time for this process, even if well-meaning friends and relatives would like us to get over it quickly.

Grieving for a child with disabilities

We need to be allowed to grieve the loss of a perfect child, and all the fantasies and dreams we had about our baby's appearance and potential. Until we have released these projections, we will not be free to accept and bond with what we may perceive as our "imperfect" child.

It is possible to suffer a loss of self-esteem, arising from the perception that our child's imperfection reflects negatively on us. Resolution includes acceptance of our baby's individual characteristics, development, and potential as separate from our own.

By accepting and showing care for the baby ourselves, and by recognizing their individual characteristics, we can learn by example to appreciate their uniqueness. Caregivers can facilitate bonding by observing when we feel ready to care for our infants. We may need encouragement to maintain open communication and an honest expression of our feelings.

It can be helpful to source information about our children's conditions and obtain referrals to support services, such as genetic counseling, professional counseling, and support groups.

Stillbirth

Our approach toward how we want to birth a baby who has died in utero may differ. Some of us may want the baby delivered immediately; others may need to hold on to our babies in the womb a while longer. Information can be sought for decisions on whether to induce labor or not.

If we had been planning a "natural birth," sometimes it is helpful to consider the option of an epidural. The numbness of an epidural may match the numbness in our hearts. It is more common for labors to be longer and slower than usual. The stage of birthing the baby may be quite difficult.

Future pregnancies

It is not unusual to feel that we never want to have more children. Or we may want to replace our lost child immediately. However, having another baby very soon may delay grief until the new birth. We may also find that it quite difficult to appreciate the new child who may not live up to the idealized image we hold in our hearts of our improperly grieved-for baby. Enough time should be set aside at your first prenatal visit to discuss the previous loss.

The following issues may need to be addressed in a subsequent pregnancy:
- Anxiety about losing the new baby may be strong.
- The last few weeks of pregnancy may be particularly long with heightened anxiety.
- The birth may re-open the wounds of loss.
- It may be more difficult to relax and accept our new babies, since we may be concerned that something awful will happen to them.

Supporting someone who has lost a child

Enormous patience is required when working with bereaved parents. By developing an attitude of allowing yourself to just "be" with them and their emotions, you can support the most powerful healing at this time. The process requires accepting that sometimes their need is simply to go over and over and over the same story, so that they might slowly allow the pain into their hearts—encouraging them not to try to change it, but to simply stay with whatever arises. Stephen Levine refers to this as a "Braille method," where people feel their way along, one moment at a time, often not knowing what the next moment will bring.

Caregiver support
- Encourage friends, family, and physicians to acknowledge the death.
- Allow them to deal with the shock in whichever way feels right for them. They may need to cry if they feel sad, or rant and rave if they feel angry.
- Let them name the child, even if she was stillborn.
- Encourage them to hold their baby. However painful this might seem at the time, it can help them to come to terms with the loss. Prepare them for this beforehand by

explaining that the baby is cold/bruised/blue, etcetera. Swaddle the baby, wipe her face, and close her eyes before presenting her to the parents. Psychiatrists have found that the relatives of those missing in action or lost in battle (those whose bodies are never recovered) have the hardest time coming to terms with their grief.

- Ask them if they would like a photo of their baby, or a snippet of hair, or a handprint—some memento for later, after the funeral.
- Parents may choose to dress their baby in her own clothes. They may wish to have their baby baptized.
- Allow parents time together on their own with their baby after the death, if they choose.
- Encourage them to have some form of funeral service.
- Provide honest, factual information. Explain as often as necessary, what happened.
- Increased flexibility of the hospital rules, if they are confined to an institution, can be of value.
- Give them reassurance, as often as they need, that it wasn't their fault that the baby died, and that there was nothing they could have done to prevent it.
- Ensure that Mom has someone to talk to about the loss. Caregivers are often busy, or feel inadequate, and her family may want to avoid the intensity of her emotions.
- If the woman has a partner who is supportive, encourage the couple to talk to one another about the death, over and over, to help with the healing.
- Do not underestimate the loss for the father.
- Help will be needed with suppression of lactation for the mother.
- Describe the emotions that they might expect to feel over the next while, and explain that unexpected emotions like self-blame and hating other people with babies is normal and natural at this time.
- Refer them to support organizations, especially a bereavement counselor.
- Let them take an active part in the organization of the funeral; it can be an opportunity to work with the grief.
- Explain to parents that it is normal to have a low libido for a while. Interest in each other and in sex will return in time.
- Ensure that parents have long-term, ongoing support. Remember that the grief will continue for a long time. Just because they might not mention it doesn't mean it has gone away. Often the support people for grieving parents forget about the episode and expect life to return to normal, long before the parents are ready for it. Remind the parents' support group to be aware of this.

Supporting someone to work through their grief

- Acknowledge the loss.
- Offer support in a specific way. Offer to visit.
- Encourage and allow communication. Let parents know you are not afraid to talk about their baby, and that you will be glad to listen. Listening is the most important thing you can do.
- Do not be afraid of periods of silence.
- Allow the expression of parent's grief. This can take the form of verbal (talking about the event, yelling, screaming), written, artistic, or physical (punching pillows, vigorous exercising) expression.
- Encourage them to limit sedative use, since it delays the grief response. However, this does not mean they should be pushed to face reality. Grief is a time when insistence on a realistic approach to life is erroneous. Rather, they may simply need gentle encouragement to endure the pain of grief, and they need some support person, who is willing to hear their story over and over, without getting bored, or feeling the need to tell them that it's time to get over it now.
- Be there for them, without trying to make it better.
- Reflect back to them, as they are talking to you, so that they are given the means to feel that you are listening to them. This is the most effective way to give them the opportunity to continue working through the story of how they are feeling. For example, after a mother has described her experience of her infant's death, you might reflect her story back to her by saying, "So what you're telling me is that you're furious at not being allowed to see your baby after she died?" This gives her the opportunity to go into greater detail, and it also lets her feel that you are truly listening to her. It may seem like repetition and may be awkward at first, but with practice, reflecting back becomes a very effective counseling tool. Don't be concerned about reflecting back incorrectly; if you do, they'll correct you.
- Redirect them to their feelings, while they are talking. "How does that feel for you?"
- Encourage them to be honest with friends and relatives about their feelings. Putting on a brave face can be stressful. Explain that they should let those people take care of them; it is not the parents' role to have to make sure their friends are feeling okay.
- Writing, perhaps in the form of a journal, can help some people work through emotions that they don't feel up to discussing with others. Writing and art are very healing forms of expression.

- It can be helpful to suggest that the parents be observant of their own and each other's physical and emotional needs. Taking exercise (even when the idea seems overwhelming), eating properly, getting adequate rest (which may be a lot more than usual), visualization, massage, and being nurtured or nurturing others can all help parents to move gradually forward in the grief process.

Misconceptions about giving support to grieving parents

- Don't think you understand or "know" what they're going through. If you haven't had a baby die under similar circumstances, you *don't* know.
- Don't tell them that you understand. The mourning period is not a time for dishonesty.
- Don't ignore the situation or neglect to offer parents sympathy and support.
- Don't offer advice too early. Often parents need someone to listen to them, so that they can work out how to get through this time by themselves. Giving advice can cut short the process of just being there for them, which is often their greatest need. If they want advice they'll usually ask for it directly.
- Don't try to make it better for them. You can't make it better. The only way to remedy the situation is for them to go through it.
- Don't get too involved in your own grief at the situation. It's not that you can't cry with them; if you do, they will be touched to know that you care so much about them. But consider that they might be needing you to play a more supportive role at this time. If a child comes to you in pain, she doesn't need you to cry with her, or to get angry at the situation; she needs you to create a safe haven for her, in which she can work through her grief. So it is with adults in pain, too.
- Don't forget the fathers. Sometimes fathers feel the need to nurture their partners and take care of all their needs when a baby is lost and may end up suppressing their own grief.
- Don't tell them your own grief stories, just to have something to say.
- Don't make light of the baby or the loss, or try to find "blessings" from the loss.

Homeopathic remedies, Bach flower remedies, aromatherapy, and massage

Physical symptoms that may arise concurrently with grief are common and include: headaches, back pain, difficulty sleeping, aching arms, loss of appetite, nausea, tension, inexplicable pains, overwhelming lethargy. More prolonged physical symptoms may manifest as shortness of breath, crushing or suffocating sensation in chest, heart palpitations, sexual difficulties, exhaustion, depressed immune system, anemia. The more severe symptoms may require referral to a GP; however, many of the physical symptoms caused by grief can be helped with homeopathic treatments.

Emotional symptoms that may be worth treating homeopathically include apathy, shock, anger, suppressed anger, grief, suppressed emotion, denial of suffering, feeling tearful, feeling tearful with difficulty, crying, crying alone, disliking consolation, feeling better for consolation, feeling depressed.

A professional homeopath, on identifying the specific emotional turmoil, will be able to offer specific remedies. Rescue Remedy and Star of Bethlehem are two Bach flower remedies that may be helpful in the initial stages.

Massage can be an appropriate form of treatment for someone who is recently bereaved, since they may be exhausted from the stress, and massage may give relief from the physical aches while also being comforting.

Aromatherapy oils that may be helpful are rose, melissa, or bergamot. Rose is indicated for those who find themselves unable to express their grief openly. Melissa is particularly valuable at the time of death; it is useful to dispel fear and regret, to bring acceptance and understanding, and to connect people to their spirituality. Bergamot has an affinity with the heart chakra, and is particularly valuable when the heart chakra is affected by grief.[121]

Relationships with our partners during the time of grieving

The stress of all our conflicting emotions can put an enormous strain on our relationships with one another, particularly as we are unlikely to deal with our grief at the same pace, or in the same way. Often couples who may have been reliant on one another for emotional support before the death of a child find that they are so busy dealing with their own emotions, they no longer have any reserves for helping their partner deal with theirs. This situation can be exacerbated if our relationships weren't particularly supportive in the first place. Counseling may be helpful to relearn how to rely on each other for emotional support. Actively grieving people cannot help one another easily.

As mothers, we may feel that our partner is not "really" grieving, or vice versa. Irritation, impatience with our own grief, and excessive worrying about the remainder of the family all are natural reactions to grief and can put strain and tension on any relationship.

Intense grief, as is usually experienced at the death of an infant, occasionally brings couples closer together, but more often, without some guidance, leaves us feeling estranged.

Siblings and grandparents

It is important to have other people around who can acknowledge our baby's siblings at this time. Siblings may not understand what is going on, especially if they are very young, but they will have to adjust to the confusion of the situation and may feel alienated. We may feel too overwhelmed by our own feelings to be capable of dealing with the emotional needs of our other children for a while.

Siblings should be told the truth about the loss, otherwise they may fantasize that they are the cause of the loss. They should be reassured that this was not their fault, and that they are loved and cared for despite everything that has occurred.

Drawing is a very good way for young children to express what they are feeling, particularly if their vocabulary is not yet developed enough to express themselves and their confusion verbally. Older children, too, often find emotional release through drawing. Children are often not allowed to give free rein to their emotions, and, therefore, may have learned to suppress their feelings from a young age.

Referral for counseling can be helpful for siblings, especially if the parents are receiving counseling. Having their own special time and attention from the counselor can help siblings feel included in the grieving process.

As a grandparent, the pain of watching a son or daughter deal with the loss of their baby can be intense. Grandparents often wish they could take on their child's grief for them, while at the same time dealing with their own loss of a grandchild.

Ina May Gaskin, in her book, *Spiritual Midwifery,* has this advice:

> There is no more helpless feeling than that one that comes when a child dies despite everyone's best efforts and prayers to keep him alive. It's a heart-breaker every time, and you don't ever get used to it. If you try to harden yourself and not feel the grief that naturally follows the death of someone who is part of your heart, you will repress that grief, and it will make you weird to do that. If you try not to feel the hurt in your mind and heart, it does not make the hurt disappear—your grief will manifest later in other ways. It's okay to cry. Grief has its own dignity. To feel it makes you telepathic with everyone else who has ever mourned, and it makes you more compassionate of others. Hold on tight to your family. Losing someone dear to you is one of the risks you take in loving anyone at all. If you keep your heart open, the rawness of the hurt will go away in time.
>
> This is how healing happens.
>
> Don't be afraid to have another child.
>
> Helping out someone else who needs it, such as a lonely old person or a child who needs special care, is a good way to help your heart to heal.

— Ina May Gaskin, American midwife, author of Spiritual Midwifery [122]

Hidden deep beneath the layers of despair, sadness, and vulnerability that grief exposes, is the emotion of tenderness, which shows itself too rarely in our world. We see it most often expressed at births, or in lovers, when our hearts are melted open, but also, perhaps more poignantly, at death, when our hearts are ripped open and shredded by death's awfulness, especially if we allow ourselves to stay true to the emotions raging through us. Tenderness implies weakness and vulnerability to pain; it expresses itself when we surrender to all that life has to offer. The word "tender" has two sources: it derives from the Latin, *tener*, meaning soft, delicate in texture or consistency; fragile; sensitive to, or easily affected by. Another derivation is from the Latin word, *tendere*, meaning to stretch. When we are stretched beyond our defences, with our deepest selves exposed, we lose our boundaries and become one with our surroundings, tender to the subtlest vibrations of the Universe.

THE PULSE OF LIFE

Chapter Eight

> " What we need, and what we love, what consoles us and what redeems us, are here each moment, already within us. It waits for us to recognize its presence. We have only to give ourselves up to it, and our one life, and all life, welcomes us into its arms. "
>
> — *John Tarrant, Zen Buddhist, psychotherapist* [123]

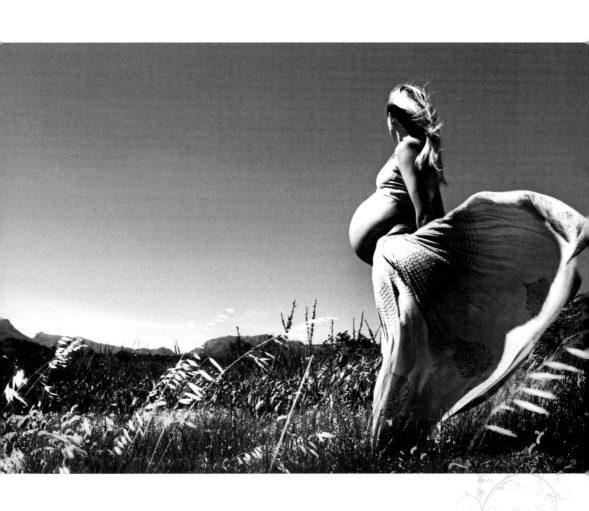

We can use the methods offered in this book for grounding us in the here and now. Life itself offers us very real opportunities to simply be present all the time. Our children are the very best teachers for demanding our presence. My youngest child used to get furious with me for constantly removing myself into myriad fantasy scenarios when he required me to be *there* with him to answer his questions and to explore life. Ani Tenzin Palmo, a calm and practical nun who spent twelve years living in a cave high up in the snowy mountains in the Himalayas, sparkles with her quality of presence. She says we take care of our outward appearance, our clothes, our hair, our homes, but we pay so little attention to our minds, which go everywhere with us and are filled with the garbage of "resentments, jealousies and frustrations going way back to childhood."[124] She says, "Suppose we all had loud-speakers attached to our minds and everyone could hear exactly what we were thinking out loud. Wouldn't everyone want to learn how to meditate and control the mind very quickly?" Mostly it is all this "junk" filling our minds that keeps us from attending to life, our births, and our babies with awareness, love, and compassion.

Birth is a metaphor for life. An extreme metaphor. There is a rhythm to life, to birth, to breathing—an inflow and an outflow. If we choose to birth naturally we have no choice but to enter into the moment of birth fully and with focused attention, taking each surge as it arises and staying present with it until its completion. The surrender that is required for birth is only a reflection of the surrender that best supports our movement back and forth through life, as we are washed by the tides of circumstance.

We are born knowing that our way back to wholeness is through our relationship with others. At birth, our consciousness is expanded into the whole—we feel one with all other beings; yet, one of our most primitive survival instincts creates a yearning for love from the others around us. Each moment of real connection has the explosive potential of an atom bomb. It emanates from a minute spark; yet, it has the potential ability to transform consciousness and the way we relate to the world. In the war-torn, violent culture of the 21st century, the human spirit is kept alive through moments of tenderness, small stories of human courage that give us hope. The woman who has such compassion for her abductors that, even though they try to rape her and threaten to kill her continuously for a terrorizing nine hours, manages to breathe in their pain and breathe out compassion for them. She has lost all instinct for survival under their threats, and all that remains is enormous empathy for the pain her attackers must have experienced for them to wish her so much harm themselves. Something about her quality of being creates a situation where they find themselves unable to rape her and, finally, unable to kill her. She is left unharmed and surprisingly untraumatized, with a story that is inspirational to those who are also living with the constant threat of violence in their lives.

Our babies are being born into this violent world, and they are protected from emotional harm by moments of pure connection. The constant plea from unborn children to their parents is for stillness and present-moment awareness of them in the weeks after birth. Monica and Paul's baby told them he wanted them to reflect on what would be taking place around them at the time of birth—not to rush into things, just to stop and pay attention. Monica said, "He wants things to be simple, not to rush, to simplify and slow down a bit and take the time to get to know him." She felt that the child was giving her a glowing energy that radiated through her eyes and head. "It's like a sense of being connected, at one with myself, with Paul, with the Universe—a harmonizing synchrony."

There is nothing to do at this time that is as important for our babies as simple attention and love. Letting go of distraction is all that is required of us.

Breathing in, inhale their baby smell.

Breathing out, softly descend into the body, meeting their gaze as fully as they meet yours.

Falling into this place of unconditional love that they offer you,

There is nowhere to go,

No one to be,

Nothing to do.

Endnotes

1   Wilson, Lois. *Midwifery Today Magazine*. August 2005.

2   Williamson, Marianne. *Return to Love*. New York: Harper Collins. 1992.

3   Rilke, Duino. Elegies. 7th Elegy.

4   Marianne Littlejohn, home-birth midwife. Cape Town. South Africa.

5   Professor Justus Hofmeyer. Author of study on labor support.

6   Susan Lees, independent midwife. Cape Town, South Africa.

7   de Mille, Agnes. Martha: *The Life and Work of Martha Graham*. New York: Random House, 1991.

8   Kornfield, Jack. *A Path with Heart*. New York: Bantam Books. 1993.

9   Trungpa, Chogyam. Shambhala, *The Sacred Path of the Warrior*. Boston, MA: Shambhala Publications. 1984.

10   Buckley, Sarah J. MD. *Ecstatic Birth*. Mothering Magazine, issue 111, March-April, 2002.

11   Blakemore, Phyllis, Sidoli, Mara. *When the Body Speaks: The Archetypes in the Body*. New York: Routledge. 2000.

12   Rachel Mendelson studied integration therapy with me in Amsterdam. I am indebted to her for her input on mythologies as they relate to birth.

13   Mauger, Benig. "Childbirth as Initiation and Transformation: The Wounded Mother." *Journal of Prenatal and Perinatal Psychology of Health*. Vol. 11 (1), 1996, pp. 17-30.

14   *Midwifery Today* magazine. November 12, 2003.

15   Jampolsky, Gerald G. *Love is Letting go of Fear*. Berkeley, CA: Celestial Arts. 1979.

16   Grof, Stanislav. *Realms of the Human Unconscious: Observations from LSD Research*. Quinn Rocks, Australia: Condor Books. 1996.

17   Janov, Arthur. *The Primal Scream. Primal Therapy. The Cure for Neurosis*. Whitefish, MT: Kessinger Publishing, LLC. 2007.

18   Wikipedia.

19   Oliver, Mary. "Wild Geese," in *Dream Work*.

20   Saint Bernard of Clairvaux. French abbot canonized in 1174.

21   Tarrant, John. *The Light Inside the Dark*. New York: Harper Collins. 1998. p. 17.

22   Campbell, Joseph, Moyers, Bill. *The Power of Myth*. New York: Anchor. 1991.

23   *Midwifery Today* magazine. Winter 2003, Number 68.

24   Biodanza, a form of dance created by Rolando Toro in Argentina, recognizes five channels of life-force energy that can be awakened through dance: Vitality, creativity, sexuality, affectivity (or relationships), and transcendence.

25   Odent, Michel. *Preventing Violence or Developing the Capacity to Love: Which Perspective? Which Investment?* Primal Health Research 2(3) Winter, 1994.

26   Laughlin, Charles D. *"Pre- and perinatal brain development and enculturation. A biogenetic structural approach."* Springer, New York. Vol. 2, Number 3, Sept 1991.

27   Verny, Thomas. *The Secret Life of the Unborn Child*. New York: Time Warner. 2006. p. 67.

28   Mauger, B. *Reclaiming the Spirituality of Birth*. Rochester, VT: Healing Arts Press. 2000. p. 51.

29   Ibid.

30   Chamberlain, D. "What Babies are teaching us about violence (Presidential address)." *Pre- and Perinatal Psychology Journal*, 10(2).

31   Verny, Thomas. *The Secret Life of the Unborn Child*. New York: Time Warner. 2006. p. 37.

32   Schwartz, L. *Bonding before Birth*. Boston, MA: Sigo Press. 1991. p. 28.

33   Ibid. p. 31-32.

34   Ibid. p. p. 33.

35   Mauger, B. *Reclaiming the Spirituality of Birth*. Rochester, VT: Healing Arts Press. 2000. p. 52.

36   Schwartz, L. *Bonding before Birth*. Boston, MA: Sigo Press. 1991. p.39 –40.

37   Ibid. p. 40.

38   Rosario N. Rozada Montemurro, "Singing Lullabies to Unborn Children: Experience in Village Vilamarxant, Spain," *Pre- and Perinatal Psychology Journal* 11, no. 1 (1996). pp 9-16.

39   Schwartz, L. *Bonding before Birth*. Boston, MA: Sigo Press. 1991. p. 34.

40   Lieberman, Michael. "Early Development of Stress and Later Behavior." *Science*, 1141(1963). p. 824.
41   Beck, M. *Expecting Adam*. London, UK: Piatkus Ltd. 2000.
42   Wildner, Kim. *Mother's Intention: How Belief Shapes Birth*. New York: Harbor Hill. 2003.
43   Cohen, Jill. *Midwifery Today*. October 29, 2003.
44   Wagner, Marsden. MD. *Midwifery Today*. February 19, 2003.
45   Shanley, Laura. Birthed five children at home, all unassisted *Midwifery Today* magazine, August 17, 2005
46   Johnson, Kenneth C. Daviss, Betty-Anne. "Outcomes of planned home births with certified professional midwives: large prospective study in North America." *BMJ* 2005;330:1416 (18 June), doi:10.1136/bmj.330.7505.1416
47   http://www.childbirthconnection.org.
48   Jensen, Katherine. *Midwifery Today* magazine. October 12, 2005.

Studies comparing Caesarean with Vaginal births

49   http:www.childbirthconnection.org/cesareanbooklet/
50   Herbert, Tennessee (1999). More than three times as many women who had had Caesarean sections (8.9 percent) than vaginal births (2.6 percent) had childbirth-related morbidities that involved **prolonged hospitalization** or **rehospitalization**.
51   Chaim, Israel. Study of **endometritis** (inflammation of the membrane lining the uterus) involving 75,947 women postpartum women. Women with fever due to known other causes were excluded. Women who had had a Caesarean section were fifteen times more likely to experience endometritis than women having vaginal births. About one in twenty-five of those who had a Caesarean section had severe infection of their abdominal wound. Women who have given birth vaginally have no abdominal wound.
52   Kacmar, (2003). A study of women having **emergency postpartum hysterectomies** within fourteen days of birth (the hysterectomies included in this study were conducted after the births, not during Caesarean sections). It excluded all women not eligible for vaginal birth (previous placenta previa, breech, three or more prior Caesarean sections) or not offered the option of vaginal birth. 79 women out of 122,025 in the study had emergency hysterectomies. Of these, 68 had delivered their babies by Caesarean section and 11 had had vaginal deliveries.
53   Lydon, Rochelle, (2000). Study of 256,795 first-time mothers giving birth to a live babies. Relative to spontaneous vaginal birth, Caesarean section was associated with an 80 percent increased risk of rehospitalization, and an instrumental vaginal birth was associated with a 30 percent increased risk for **rehospitalization**. Hospital readmission diagnoses: uterine infection (27.0 percent) pp hemorrhage (21.6 percent), gallbladder disease (18.8 percent), genitourinary complications (11.7 percent), breast infection (10.9 percent), obstetrical surgical wounds (8.2 percent), mental health (6.2 percent) cardiopulmonary complications (6.1 percent) thromboembolic complications (3.7 percent), pelvic injury (includes disruption of perineal wound, pelvic hematoma, thrombozed hemorrhoids, fistularectal abscess) (3.1 percent), appendicitis (2.9 percent).
54   **Maternal Mortality Rate**
       Study 1. Schuitemaker, van Roosmalen, Dekker, et al. Reported a Maternal Mortality Rate of 4/100,000 for vaginal delivery and of 53/100,000 for Caesarean section in the Netherlands during the ten-year period of 1983–1992. Based on their data, they calculated a risk of 28/100,000 for the effects of Caesarean section alone. Of the deaths after Caesarean section, ten were judged directly due to the surgery and four to a complication of anesthesia, and in sixteen cases, Caesarean section contributed to death (ex. embolism or sepsis). Study 2. Harper (2003) Study based on maternal mortality comparison of Caesarean compared to vaginal births. The study looked at 118 pregnancy-related deaths with live birth within one year of birth ascertained from database linkages, compared to controls of 3697 randomly selected births: 35.9/100,000 women died after Caesarean sections. 9.2/100,000 women died after vaginal births. Adjusted Odds Ratios were controlled for medical complications, pre-term delivery, and age.
55   **Pain at incision site**
       Study 1. Declercq (2002) US. 7 percent of mothers who had had Caesarean sections still reported pain at incision site six months post-operatively. Study 2. Fisher. (1997) Australia. Study on post partum pain relief. 100 percent of

women who had a Caesarean section required pain relief. 11 percent of women who birthed vaginally required pain relief.

56 **Women's feelings about their birth experience**

Study 1. Jolly (1999) UK. Study based on a questionnaire sent to women five years post-birth. Those who reported a bad experience: 22.4% of Caesarean mothers. 9.5% of mothers who had a vaginal delivery. Those who reported a disappointing experience: 49% of Caesarean mothers, 18% of mothers who had a vaginal delivery. Study 2. DiMatteo (1996) Meta analysis of forty-three studies of psychosocial outcomes of Caesarean section published between 1979 and 1993. The analysis excluded mothers and babies with health problems. Caesarean section was found to be a powerful predicator for dissatisfaction with birth.

57 DiMatteo (1996) Meta analysis of forty-three studies of **psychosocial outcomes** of Caesarean section published between 1979 and 1993. The analysis excluded mothers and babies with health problems. The analysis found that fewer Caesarean-sectioned mothers initiate play. They had a less positive evaluation of their babies and experienced less positive feelings for their babies.

58 Towner, (1999). 583,340 live-born singleton infants of first-time mothers, California, 1992–1994. **Neonatal death**. Four times as many babies died before discharge after Caesarean deliveries than after spontaneous vaginal births. Data were not adjusted for potential confounding variables.

59 Kolås, T. (MD.) Saugstad, O (MD. PhD.) Daltveit, AK. (PhD.) Nilsen, ST. (MD. PhD). Øian, P. (MD. PhD). American Journal of Obstetrics & Gynecology (2007) 195: 1538-43 **Transfer to Neonatal ICU**: A planned Caesarean delivery doubled both the rate of transfer to the neonatal intensive care unit and the risk for pulmonary disorders, compared with a planned vaginal delivery.

60 Annibale, (1995). South Carolina. Community center and medical hospital. **Respiratory Distress Syndrome**. Study of 10871 Vaginal births and 1369 Caesarean-section births. Women with pregnancy complications were excluded. The study found that Caesarean delivery before onset of labor is the main factor for Respiratory Distress Syndrome. Four times as many Caesarean section as spontaneous vaginal delivery babies had dangerously low five-minute Apgar scores of between 0-3.

61 **Breast-feeding problems**

Study 1. Di Matteo (1996) Meta-analysis of nine studies. Fewer mothers who had had Caesareans breast-fed their babies than mothers who birthed their babies vaginally. Unplanned Caesarean sections had poorer breast-feeding outcomes than planned ones. Study 2 Dewey (2003) California. Study found an increased risk for delayed onset of milk production with Caesarean-section mothers. 3. Ever-Haldani, 1994. 8486 Israeli women whose previous pregnancy resulted in a child who lived at least one year: 80.3% of mothers who delivered vaginally initiated breast-feeding, whilst only 59% of mothers who had had a Caesarean section did so.

62 **Subsequent Caesarean risks**

1. Infertility

Study 1. Hemminki (1996) Eight cohort studies comparing subsequent reproduction after Caesarean section with a control group with no previous Caesarean section. This group of studies found that there is a reduced rate of fertility among women with prior Caesarean-section births. Study 2. Jolly, 1999. A study of parents who tried but didn't succeed to fall pregnant for subsequent children. The group of women were studied five years after their previous birth. Double the number of women who failed to conceive had had a previous Caesarean section compared to women who had had a previous vaginal delivery. Study 3. Murphy, 2002. UK. 14,541 women in this study showed there was an increased rate of sub-fertility among women who had had previous Caesarean sections as compared to women who had delivered vaginally. 11.8% as compared to 7.2%.

2. Reduced desire for further children

Jolly (1999) UK. A study of women five years after their previous birth who were questioned about their feelings of having another child: 26.1% of women who had had a previous Caesarean were frightened to have another child, as compared to 10% of their counterparts who had delivered vaginally. 19% of the Caesarean group felt they couldn't go through childbirth again, while only 5% of the NVD (normal vaginal delivery) group felt similarly.

3. Ectopic pregnancy

Hemminki, 1996. Study found there was an increased likelihood of a subsequent ectopic pregnancy (pregnancy where the embryo implants in the fallopian tube leading from the ovary to the womb, rather than in the womb itself) in women who had had one or more previous Caesarean deliveries.

63   Miller (1997) Los Angeles, 1985–1994. 155,670 births in Los Angeles, 62 cases of histologically confirmed **placenta accreta** (placenta unable to dislodge from uterine wall after birth) and 590 cases of **placenta previa** (placenta attaching over the cervix or mouth of womb, instead of to uterine wall). As per the graph, this study found that a previous Caesarean created an increased risk of placenta previa and of placenta accreta when compared to women who hadn't had a previous Caesarean section. This risk increased exponentially with subsequent Caesarean sections.

64   Rageth (1999) Study of 255,453 women who had had one or more previous birth, including 29,046 with a prior Caesarean section. Switzerland, 1983–1996 This study found that women who had had a previous Caesarean section had a significantly increased risk of: **bleeding in pregnancy with placenta previa, bleeding in pregnancy with placental abruption, abruption during labor, uterine rupture, emergency hysterectomy, ileus,** (intestinal obstruction) **thromboembolic complications, perinatal death of baby** Only maternal mortality did not reach significance.

65   Cardwell CR, Stene LC, Jones G, et al. Caesarean section is associated with an increased risk of **childhood-onset type 1 diabetes mellitus:** Meta-analysis of observational studies. Department of Epidemiology and Public Health, Queen's University, Belfast. Analysis of twenty studies demonstrated a 20% increase in the risk of childhood-onset type 1 diabetes after Caesarean section delivery that could be explained by known confounders.

66   Sakala, Carol (PhD) http://www.childbirthconnection.org

67   Bateman, Chris. "C-section protocol: Rendering unto Caesar." *South African Medical Journal.* October 2004. Vol 94, No. 10.

68   Gaskin, Ina May. *Spiritual Midwifery.* Book Publishing Company. 1979.

69   Shakespeare, William. *Hamlet.* Polonius' advice to his son Laertes.

70   Rinehart, Heidi. (MD) as quoted in Gaskin, Ina May. Ina May's Guide to Childbirth. New York: Bantam Books. 2003.

71   Chödrön, Pema. *Start Where You Are: A Guide to Compassionate Living.* Boston, MA: Shambhala Publications. 1994.

72   Georgia O'Keeffe, American artist 1887-1996.

73   Thich Nhat Hanh. *Present Moment, Wonderful Moment.* Berkeley, CA: Parallax Press. p. 32.

74   Antoine de Saint-Exupery. *The Little Prince.* Fort Washington, PA: Harvest Books. 2000.

75   Buckley, Sarah. *Midwifery Today* magazine. May 14, 2003.

76   Chödrön, Pema. *The Places that Scare You: A Guide to Fearlessness in Difficult Times.* Boston, MA: Shambhala Classics. 2002.

77   Arnaud Desjardins, formerly a well known film-maker, is an eminent French spiritual teacher.

78   Field, T. Hernandez-Reif, M. Taylor, S. Quintino, 0. Burman, I. (1997). *Journal of Psychosomatic Obstetrics and Gynecology*, 18, 286-291.

79   Ibid.

80   Field, T. Hernandez-Reif, M. Hart, S. Theakston, H. Schanberg, S. Kuhn, C. Burman, I. (1999) "Pregnant women benefit from massage therapy." *Journal of Psychosomatic Obstetrics and Gynecology*, 19, pp. 31-38.

81   Keating, Kathleen. *Hug Therapy Book.* Center City, MN: Hazelden Publishers. 1995.

82   Kennell, John H. (MD) pediatrician, author and "father" of the modern doula movement.

83   Jung, C.G. *Alchemical Studies*, Vol 15, 1954. pp. 470.

84   Tarrant, John. *The Light Inside the Dark.* New York: Harper Collins, 1998. p. 232.

85   Many of the ideas for birth ceremonies were taken from http://www.blessingway.net.

86   Buckley, Sarah J. MD. "Ecstatic Birth." *Mothering Magazine*, issue 111, March-April 2002.

87   Sagady, Mayri. Midwifery Today magazine. December 11, 2002.

88   Goer, Henci. http://parenting.ivillage.com/pregnancy/plabor/0,,bxkm-p,00.html.

89   Sogyal, Rinpoche. *The Tibetan Book of Living and Dying.* New York: Harper Collins. 1992.

90   Verny, Thomas. *The Secret Life of the Unborn Child.* New York: Time Warner. 2006. p. 17.

91   Ibid. p. 36.

92   Ibid. p. 37.

93   Cullen, C. Field, T. Escalona, A. Hartshorn, K. (2000) "Father-infants interactions are enhanced by massage therapy." *Journal of Early Child Development and Care*. Vol 164, pp. 41-47.

94   The Royal College of Obstetricians and Gynaecologists guidelines - Induction of Labor. http://www.nice.org.uk/pdf/inductionoflabourrcogrep.pdf.

95   Darwin, Erasmus. (Charles Darwin's grandfather). *Zoonomia*, 1801.

96   *CIA, The World Fact Book, 2006*: https://www.cia.gov/cia/publications/factbook/fields/2091.html.

97   Morley, GM. "Cord Closure: Can Hasty Clamping Injure the Newborn?" OBG Management (July 1998) 29-36.

98   Ultee, K. Swart, J. Van der Deure, H. Lasham, C. van Baar,A. "Delayed cord clamping in preterm infants delivered at 34 to 36 weeks gestation: A randomized controlled trial." *BMJ*. 2007.

99   http://www.empoweredchildbirth.com/articles/birth/noclamp.html.

100 Leboyer, Frederick. *Birth Without Violence*. Rochester, VT: Healing Arts Press. Revised edition 2002.

101 Wilson, Lois. "American midwife." Excerpt taken from *Midwifery Today* magazine.

102 Chuang-tzu, Taoist Chinese sage and philosopher, 400 BCE.

103 Kornfield, Jack. *After the Ecstasy, the Laundry*. New York: Bantam. 2001.

104 Eicho Zenrinkushu was compiled by Eicho (1429-1504), a disciple of Secco of Myoshinji. The items (four thousand in all) are collected from about two hundred books, including various Zen writings.

105 http://www.kangaroomothercare.com/ref_oprefs.htm.

106 Larimer, Krisanne. Article on Kangaroo Care Benefits. http://www.prematurity.org/baby/kangaroo.html.

107 *The Lancet*, 1998, 352:1115.

108 Field, T. (1988). "Stimulation of preterm infants". *Pediatrics in Review*, 10, pp. 149-15.

109 Bergman NJ, Linley LL, Fawcus SR. "Randomized controlled trial of maternal-infant skin-to-skin contact from birth versus conventional incubator for physiological stabilization in 1200g to 2199g newborns." Acta Paediatr (2004) 93. pp. 779-785.

110 Northrup, Christiane. (MD) *Women's Bodies, Women's Wisdom*. New York: Bantam. 2002.

111 Oski, Frank. Retired editor, *Journal of Paediatrics*.

112 Field, T. Grizzle, N. Scafidi, F. Abrams, S. Richardson, S. Kuhn, C. Shanberg, S.(1996). Study on "Massage therapy for infants of depressed mothers." *Journal of Infant Behavior and Development*. Vol 19. pp. 109-114.

113 St. Catherine of Siena. Daniel Ladinsky. *Love Poems from God*. New York: Penguin Compass. 2002.

114 Blakemore, Phyllis, Sidoli, Mara. *When the Body Speaks: The Archetypes in the Body*. New York: Routledge. 2000.

115 Gibran, Kalil. *The Prophet*. New York: Alfred A. Knopf. 1946. p. 35.

116 Hart, Hilary. "The Unknown She. Eight Faces of an Emerging consciousness," interview with Harvey Andrew. The Golden Sufi Center. 2003.

117 Simos, Bertha. *A Time to Grieve*. Family Service Association of America. 1979. pp. 38-39.

118 Levine, Stephen. *Healing into Life and Death*. New York: Anchor Books. 1987. Pp. 109, 110.

119 Kornfield, Jack. *A Path with Heart*. New York: Bantam Books. 1993. p. 47.

120 *Varneys Midwifery Manual*. New York: Jones & Bartlett Publishers, Inc. 2003.

121 Davis, Patricia. *Subtle Aromatherapy*. London: Random House. 1991.

122 Gaskin, Ina May. *Spiritual Midwifery*. Summertown, TN: The Book Publishing Company. 1990. p. 273.

123 Tarrant, John. *The Light Inside the Dark*. New York: Harper Collins. 1998. p. 239.

124 Palmo, Ani Tenzin. "Discovering Basic Sanity," a talk given in Tasmania. July 2000.

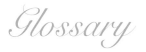

Glossary

Adrenaline – (Epinephrine in the US) When the sympathetic nervous system sends a stress message to the adrenal glands, they respond with the production of adrenaline. Adrenaline is a hormone that causes the flight, fright, fight response to stressful situations.

Amniotic fluid – A transparent, albuminous fluid surrounding the baby in the amniotic sac within the womb. Amniotic fluid protects the baby from injury, maintains the temperature inside the womb, and prevents the amniotic sac from sticking to the skin of the growing fetus.

Anterior fontanelle – A fontanelle is an anatomical feature on an infant's skull. Fontanelles are soft spots on a baby's head that, during birth, enable the bony plates of the skull to flex, allowing the child's head to pass through the birth canal. The ossification of the bones of the skull causes the fontanelle to close over by a child's second birthday. The closures eventually form part of the sutures of the skull. The much larger, diamond-shaped anterior fontanelle, where the two frontal and two parietal bones join, is the soft spot just to the fore of the crown of the head.

Archetype – An unconscious idea, pattern of thought, or image that is universally applicable to the condition of human experience or to the psyche.

Augmentation – The artificial stimulation of labor with drugs, usually pitocin or misoprostol, to increase the number and intensity of contractions during labor.

Aum – is a mystical or sacred syllable in Hinduism. It is a sacred sound representing Brahman, the impersonal Absolute—omnipotent, omnipresent, and the source of all manifest existence. It is thought to be the original sound.

Autonomic nervous system (ANS) – Functions subconsciously to maintain homeostasis in the human body, including heart rate, digestion, respiration rate, salivation, perspiration, micturition (passing urine), and erection. Whereas most of its actions are involuntary, some ANS functions work in tandem with the conscious mind, such as breathing.

Birth attendant – A professional birth companion whose role is to provide emotional support during labor and to help a woman trust in her bodies' ability to give birth.

Cervix – The neck of the womb. The cervix is the opening at the base of the womb that dilates to ten centimeters in diameter during labor to allow the baby to pass through it and down through the birth canal.

Chakra – Part of the human energy field, the word "chakra" literally translates as "wheel" or "disk" and refers to spinning spheres of bioenergetic activity emanating from the major nerve ganglia branching forward from the spinal column. The major chakras in the human body comprise seven energy wheels, spanning from the base of the spine to the crown of the head. The major chakras correlate with basic states of consciousness.

Chi – Life-force energy, or vital energy, pervading all matter, animate and inanimate. Chi is scientifically measurable. Living organisms emit energy vibrations at a frequency of between three hundred and two thousand nanometers.

Dilation – The term used to describe how advanced a woman is in labor by checking on how far her cervix has opened. It must stretch from closed to about ten centimeters in diameter in order to let the baby pass through it, into the vagina, and out into the world.

Doula – Greek for "slave." A common term used to describe a professional labor attendant.

Electronic fetal heartmonitor – A machine that measures the fetal heart beat to denote fetal well-being.

Endorphin – An opiate produced by the brain that causes sensations of analgesia and of well-being.

Entrega – Spanish word which doesn't have an acceptable English equivalent. Its direct translation is "submission" or "delivery," however, in Spanish it is used in the context of letting go into the flow of life in a voluptuous surrender to all that is.

Epidural anaesthesia – Regional anaesthesia that blocks pain in a particular region of the body. Epidurals block the nerve impulses from the lower spinal segments resulting in decreased sensation in the lower half of the body. Epidural medications fall into a class of drugs called local anesthetics. They are often delivered in combination with opioids or narcotics to decrease the required dose of local anesthetic. The "epidural space" is found outside the dural membrane surrounding the brain and spinal cord below the L5 vertebra. Epidural anaesthesia is the most popular means of drug relief for pain during labor.

Estrogen – The word derives from the Greek *oistros* meaning "mad desire" and *gennan* meaning "to produce." Estrogen is the female hormone that induces the development of female sexual characteristics and the cyclical periods of estrus, when the body is at its most fertile. The hormones are produced by the ovaries.

Fetus – The unborn child.

Hara – Japanese equivalent of the Chinese term tan tien. An energy center about four centimeters (1.5 inches) below the navel in the middle of the body, that is known as our center of gravity and is the point martial artists focus on to stay grounded, focused, and centered.

Harmonic resonance – Correlates to the feeling of "being in the zone." A sense of oneness or feeling at ease in one's surroundings. The underlying feeling of love that pervades everything when we feel safe enough to drop the barriers we put up to protect ourselves from the world.

Homeostasis – the ability to regulate the internal environment of the body so as to maintain a stable, constant condition.

HypnoBirthing – Deep relaxation techniques for labor and birth.

Induction - The artificial stimulation of labor with drugs, usually pitocin or misoprostol, to start and maintain contractions until the baby is born.

Integration therapy – Individualized work of identifying and releasing emotional traumas, which are held in the body and which negatively impact the way we react to the external circumstances of our lives.

Limbic brain – Limbic derives from the Latin word meaning "border." The limbic brain is the first part of the brain formed in the embryo. It is our ancient brain and manages hormones in animals and in man. It is involved with emotional responses and with memory, which it manages by integrating emotional states with stored memories of physical sensations.

Meconium – Is the first stool passed by a baby at birth. It is thick, black, and tarry in consistency. If a baby passes meconium before birth or during labor, it often indicates a period of fetal distress, often due to their mother's exposure to physiological or psychological stress.

Oxytocin – Pituitary hormone that stimulates uterine surges in labor, the let-down reflex for breast-feeding and orgasm during sexual activity. Emotionally it correlates to a feeling of love.

Perineum – The external region between the vulva and the anus constituting the pelvic floor.

Placental barrier - The semipermeable layer of tissue in the placenta that serves as a selective membrane to substances passing from maternal to fetal blood.

Primal brain – hypothalamus and limbic brain. Directs our instinctual behavior.

Posterior fontanelle – See anterior fontanelle. The smaller posterior fontanelle is the soft spot on a baby's skull found at the top point of the back of the skull.

Progesterone – Is a hormone produced by the ovaries and the placenta. It prepares the lining of the uterus to receive a fertilized egg and to maintain a pregnancy.

Subtle energy – (Chi) Beyond the physical body, there exists a subtle energy field of a higher vibrational frequency. Our subtle energy field makes up our "aura."

Tan tien – Chinese equivalent of the Japanese term hara. An energy center about four centimeters (1.5 inches) below the navel in the middle of the body, that is known as our center of gravity and is the point martial artists focus on to stay grounded, focused, and centered.

Testosterone – Male hormone produced by the adrenal glands responsible for secondary sexual characteristics in males and erections. Emotionally associated with masculine characteristics of aggression, protection, and strength.

Toning – Toning is the creation of extended vocal sounds on a single vowel in order to experience the sound and its effects in other parts of the body.

Transition – The final stage of the dilation phase of labor, prior to birthing the baby through the birth canal.

Universal energy – The "sea" of cosmic consciousness, that penetrates and underlies all physical manifestation.

Vacuum extraction – Assisted delivery of the fetus during vaginal birth, using a suction cup applied to the head of the fetus.

Water birth – A method of giving birth, that involves immersion in warm water. The effect of buoyancy that deep-water immersion creates allows the mother to move spontaneously during labor. This easy ability to move helps open the pelvis, allowing the baby to descend. Benefits of water birth include pain relief during labor for the mother and possibly a less traumatic birth experience for the baby.

Wu wei – Chinese expression describing a sense of flowing with the currents of life without resistance.

Web links

www.mamabamba.co.za – Website for our center in Cape Town, which offers classes and individual therapies to support parents on their incredible journey through birth and into parenting.

www.birthworks.co.za - South African Website offering locally available birthing resources, including midwives, birth attendants, birth pool, and birth equipment rentals and an online advice column.

www.gentlebirth.org – An accessible and informative directory for midwives and parents on birth related issues from a holistic paradigm.

www.biodanza.co.za - Biodanza is a form of dance for awakening vitality and life force. It is a fusion of music, movement, and emotion aimed at improving the quality of relationships and creating general well-being and happiness.

www.hypnobirthing.com - HypnoBirthing® is a unique method of relaxed, natural childbirth education, enhanced by self-hypnosis techniques.

www.kangaroomothercare.com - 44 articles and studies on "kangaroo care."

www.birthworks.org/site/primal-health-research – Dr. Michel Odent's data-bank on birth-related studies. It explores correlations between the "primal period" (from conception until the first birthday) and health in later life.

www.childbirthconnection.org - Statistics on research comparing modes of birth. See: http://www.childbirthconnection.org/cesareanbooklet/

www.blessingways.net – Ideas for birth ceremonies.

www.parenting.ivillage.com/pregnancy/plabor/0,,bxkm-p,00.html - Are you really in labor? Seven questions to help you know for sure.

www.miami.edu/touch-research/research.htm - Touch Research Institute at the University of Miami. Over a 100 different published studies illustrating the benefits of touch and massage. Many of these are focused on perinatal groups and on behavioral development of infants.

www.pushedbirth.com - A US-based Website encouraging natural birth and describing the drawbacks of birth that is medically over managed.

www.babycentre.co.uk – Easy-to-access search engine for birth-related issues.

www.dona.org/resources/research.php – The DONA (Doulas Of North America) Website lists many of the studies that have been undertaken researching the impact of doulas on birth.

Acknowledgments

This book is a blend of ideas and inspiration from almost everybody I know. Many people directly contributed with generous offerings of time, encouragement, and wisdom: Rachel Mendelson brought her deep understanding and advice about archetypes; Linda Glynn added practical breast-feeding advice; Ken Findlay offered patient hours teaching me the subtleties of my computer's brain; Dr. Carol Sakala was helpful with feedback and generous with her research on Caesarean section studies; Bill Petrie, Marlies Van Boxtel, Sister Châu Nghiêm, Donal Creedon, Gilly Barton, and Justine Evans read the manuscript, or parts thereof, and gave me detailed feedback. Thanks, too, to my dear friends Justine, Kate Spreckley, and Sarah Heinamann for all the fun hours spent creating Mamabamba together.

Lovely Zann Hoad had a vision for our book that was so similar to mine. She just fell into my life, added a wonderful interview about her Caesarean sections, and then proceeded to become my South African publisher in such an easy and natural way.

Nikki Rixon, photographer and meditation friend, accompanied me to classes, to clients, and to births at all hours of the night, in order to take the beautiful photographs that grace this book.

Adele Sherlock, graphic designer, is a true craftswoman. It was a pleasure to sit alongside her as she worked with such meticulous care on the layout.

Strong women role models over the years who have informed my outlook on life have been my aunt Pat Burgess, my integration therapy teacher Marlies Van Boxtel, and from way back, ceramicist Lesley-Ann Hoets.

My midwifery colleagues and friends, Elise Kimmons and Althea Seaver, Martha Mothibe, and Evelyn Bender, Sue Lees, Ciska Van Straten, Karen Clarke, Marianne Littlejohn, and Natasha Stadler all gave me much encouragement, through trusting me and through teaching me so much about birth. And, of course, Ruth Pfau also fits into this acknowledgment, even though she's an obstetrician, not a midwife.

Thanks to the people who have taught me to trust my own body, since I spend so much time teaching pregnant women that this is the most important thing they can do for their labors—Carolina Churba, Biodanza teacher; François Moller, supportive dance friend; and Rebecca Smith who, bless her for her patience, is teaching me to sing!

Let me not forget my friends, who laugh and play and cry with me. Your list became so long and unwieldy that I decided to write you in invisible ink and place you in parentheses. If you wonder if you're there or not, you are [. . . . . . .].

Thanks are due to all my clients, who are a constant source of inspiration and who have been so generous with interviews, with feedback, and most of all with their birthing wisdom. I especially want to thank Patty Hamann, Janet Steer, Myra Miller, and Claudi Paitaki for their help. Thanks, too, to those wonderful women who participated in interviews for the book, even though they hadn't been my clients. Particular mention must go to Andrée Eva Bosch, for her courage in writing her story about losing her baby.

I would like to acknowledge my spiritual teachers. They are the guides who show me the way to negotiate my path through my life: Thich Nhat Hanh, Kittisaro, Thanissara, and Norma Milanovich.

Finally, my thanks go to my parents, John and Bob, for thinking that I'm "wonderful" and to Charlie Sheldon, best friend, ex-husband, and father of our children, for his support from both near and far over the years. And to our kids, Rory, Maf and Nix, for having wide-open, independent minds and wide-open, generous hearts.

Index